Romancing
The
Stove

A PRACTICAL GUIDE
TO A LIFELONG CELEBRATION
OF EATING FOR HEALTH

Samahria Ramsen

DISCLAIMER

There is no claim that information contained herein can be or should be used for any health problem. It is presented only as a form of knowledge from Ayurveda. This book is not intended to treat, or prescribe. The information contain herein is in no way to be considered as a substitute for consultation with a licensed health-care professional.

Published by Omnilux® Communications Inc.
Printed and bound in Canada

Cover design by Viswajit John Inglis
Author photograph by Jacob Katsman

Library of Congress Cataloguing-in-Publication Data is available upon request.
Ramsen, Samahria.
Romancing The Stove: a practical guide to a lifelong celebration of eating for health.

ISBN 0-9699078-2-6   Price: $19.95

1. Health is Wealth.
2. Art Of Living;
3. Joy Of Cooking And Eating.

DEDICATION

Dedicated to my Eternal Teacher,
Sri Tulshi.
May the ballads of his wisdom and kindness
be sung all over the world.

CONTENTS

INTRODUCTION
PUT SOME ECSTASY IN YOUR EATING

PART ONE
PRELUDE TO ROMANCE

PART TWO
OVERTURE TO THE CREATION

PART THREE
CREATING WEALTH

PART FOUR
CREATING ROMANCE

Appreciation

Let me express my feelings of love and gratitude to the following people:

Viswajit John Inglis and Madhabi Inglis for helping me in editing the manuscript, designing the cover for this book as well as testing and enjoying the recipes.

Satyajit Davies for proofreading and revelling in the recipes. Aditi Patricia Walsh for proofreading support and making the recipes a part of her life.

I also thank all the members of The International Society Of Spiritual Understanding for promoting and enjoying the Romancing The Stove method of living, cooking and eating, for their courage and commitment to a new world order, to a vision that transcends all limitations.

I am forever grateful to my mother and my beloved sister for being there for me and my children Jacob and Elina for brightening my life.

Finally, to the most important person of all - you, my reader for your effort to change your lifestyle and become a happier and healthier person by using this book. Together we will make a difference!

INTRODUCTION

PUT SOME ECSTASY IN YOUR EATING

Who Said Health Food Has To Be Blah?
Try This For Size

While vegetarianism is catching on in the Western world it is still considered by many to be part of an off-the-wall lifestyle practised by "new agers" and by those who are unable to eat meat. However, recent gains in the popularity of adopting this diet would suggest that the population of vegetarians is growing by leaps and bounds.

We are not trying to preach vegetarianism, nor do we wish to be associated with what might be considered fanatical or faddist approaches to eating food. The purpose of this book is:

a) To introduce the reader to ecstatic eating and to provide a basis for a healthy and happy life.

b) To show the aspiring vegetarian that meat, chicken or fish will not be missed.

c) To dispel the myth that the vegetarian diet does not have enough protein to promote good health. Consider such large and powerful warm-blooded animals as the elephant, the horse, the bull and the cow who prosper on a strictly vegetarian diet. The protein they require is derived from grasses and grains that are their principal source of food. We do not need to rob them of their lives in order to appropriate their protein, because with the right balance of plant food, which contains essential amino acids, we can obtain all the protein we need. Dairy products help round out our source of health giving foods. Somewhere between protein over-consumption and protein deficiency there is a balance. Any doctor worth his/her salt will tell you that too much protein is not good for you, and that the proper amount of daily protein intake is essential for health.

d) To show that by becoming a vegetarian, your social life need not be adversely affected. You can enjoy eating and be a vegetarian too.

The author used to eat raw vegetables for dinner every day until she came to the conclusion that there wasn't much enjoyment in this practice. She does empathize with those who think it is a pain to be a vegetarian, in their mistaken belief that they are restricted to raw or partially cooked vegetables, bland tofu and lentils on a daily basis.

She learned the authentic, nutritious and tasteful vegetarian cooking contained in Romancing The Stove, from her teacher, who comes from a long line of Masters originating in the foothills of the Himalayas. Under his guidance she has discovered the power and romance of food preparation and eating.

Since the body is a temporary harbour for the soul, it must be kept clean and in good order. What is good for the body is essential in helping us to realize the soul.

Cooking is not a daily event to be dispensed with as quickly as possible. The author has learned from her teacher that cooking can be the beginning of Self Romance and a form of meditation, as well as a relief from stress. Romance with the Self or the Soul is ultimately the true romance.

In Romancing The Stove the author presents the reader with her meditations in the form of recipes. It is important to realize that each dish is part of the romance and is named appropriately for a specific mood or occasion. Get into the spirit of each name while you prepare the food. The name itself will suggest what the recipe, when followed, may do for you and will help you to understand the effects of each dish on your mind and body. These recipes are the keys to health and energy.

The author cannot emphasize enough how important it is to enter into the spirit of the name of each dish while preparing, cooking and eating the food. Consider making a personal menu using these exotic names when you are romancing or entertaining. Imagine offering your family "Heavens Hash Brown" with "Warm Affection" and "A Date with The Taste Buds" for lunch. Make each meal a celebration: an offering to the body for housing your spirit.

PART ONE

PRELUDE TO ROMANCE

CHAPTER 1

WHY ROMANCING THE STOVE ?

Romancing The Stove is your guide to the discovery of the real joy of cooking and eating. Make a date with your taste buds for dancing and romancing. Nourish and rejuvenate every cell of your body; take yourself on a prolonged fun-filled picnic.

You will discover that cooking does not have to be boring. It can be exciting. Cooking is not hard work. It is easy and enjoyable. Cooking is meditation. Cooking is creative. Cooking is love.

This book is not just another cookbook. This book is based on the Vedic principles and philosophy of the ancient science of India, Ayurveda, "The Science of Life", brought to us straight from the Himalayas by Sri Tulshi. He teaches that every cell of the body has consciousness and that food is meant to nourish these cells. When you cook, the consciousness of every cell feels love and gives eternal love back to you. It creates harmony, brings health, wealth and romance.

It is through cell consciousness that all actions are performed. Through the food we eat we can give a direct suggestion to the thirty trillion cells of our body that we care for them. They in turn, care for us. Cells are like children watching their mother cooking their favourite dishes. This is how the union, or yoga of cooking and eating takes place to bring you health, happiness and wealth.

Sri Tulshi says: "Wealth without a healthy body is poverty. Your first step to riches is through "Wealth food", for Health Is Wealth. When you eat you feed God. When you cook you cook for God. Food itself is an expression of Divine Consciousness".

The first step in Romancing The Stove is to master the art of cooking and eating as a means to enhance your romance and to live a joyful life. One important factor in attaining your goal is to eat the natural way.

What Is The Real Purpose Of Eating?

The whole purpose of eating is to have a healthy body. Your body is a marvellous instrument that is sustained by food. According to the Master: "It is the universe in microcosm with the stomach as its central star. What you put in the stomach will affect your universe directly."

The function of the body is to be a proper vehicle for the spirit whose nature is bliss. Your goal is to reach out, touch excellence and realize unity. What does this have to do with the joy of eating? Everything! But first, let us find out more about our body.

The Mystery Of The Body

In this modern age we have sent probes into outer space and danced on the moon, but there are many mysteries of the body, mind and soul about which we know very little.

Our body is like the universe. It contains all the ingredients needed to produce another body. How is this accomplished? With all the accelerated advancement in this world of ours no scientist can claim to know precisely, in all its complexity, how another body is made.

Modern medicine and science is only confirming what the ancients knew about the connection between food, cooking and health. In those long-ago-times there were no hospitals, plagues or epidemics. A healthy and a beautiful body was a natural occurrence, because in the old-world people lived naturally. Today, leading a balanced life and eating the right food properly prepared can go a long way towards promoting happiness, alertness and longevity.

Romancing The Stove intends to:
1. Acquaint you with eating the natural way.
2. Show you step by step, how to sustain your body and live a life of harmony and balance.
3. Give you exciting recipes which will contribute toward your eating enjoyment and bodily health.
4. Build a sound body which is a suitable home for a happy mind and a joyful spirit.
5. Suggest that a healthy body, a happy mind and a joyful spirit can take you on a journey to the land of your dreams and bring you wealth and success in your everyday life.

Come, let us take the second step in Romancing The Stove and find out more about the food we eat.

A FEW QUICK QUESTIONS ANSWERED

You Must Have These Answers
Otherwise You Are Eating Blindly

"The essence of all beings is Earth.
The essence of the Earth is Water.
The essence of Water is plants.
The essence of plants is the Human being"

Chandogya Upanishad 1.1.2

Can vegetarian food give you enough protein?

Yes indeed, you will get enough protein from vegetarian food. These foods include grains, beans, fruits, vegetables, nuts, herbs, spices and milk products. They contain all the necessary ingredients for a long, happy and healthy life.

Proteins are the most important nutrients for our body. They are necessary for the rejuvenation of body tissues and the formation of strong fibres which hold the skeleton together. They also form antibodies which prevent disease. They regulate and coordinate the functions of the body.

Too much protein, as well as too little, is damaging to health. Eating too much protein can be the cause of various diseases. It destroys the function of the liver and kidneys and affects bone demineralization. Excess protein in the body turns into carbohydrates and accumulates as fat. It promotes obesity, high blood pressure and heart disease.

What Is Protein?

Protein is a molecule made of small building blocks called amino acids. There are 22 different kinds of amino acids in our body, 9 of which the body does not make on its own. These 9 are called essential amino acids because they must be taken from food. It is very important to have all these 9 amino acids at the same time in your meal to produce a complete protein.

All animal proteins are made from plant proteins. Those amino acids that come from rice and beans are exactly the same as the amino acids that come from beef or chicken.

How do you combine foods which will provide enough protein in your diet?

It is easy. Each day eat one of the following combinations:

- Grains and legumes.

- Milk products plus rice and vegetables.

- Vegetables with grain or rice.

- Soybeans.

What is Cholesterol?

Cholesterol comes from the Greek word "cholesterin", which means "chole"-bile and "stereos"-stiff, solid. Natural cholesterol is produced mainly in the liver as required. It is used to help digestion, build cell membranes and sex hormones. It is delivered to the appropriate cells by the bloodstream.

Your body makes exactly the right amount of cholesterol you need to build all necessary hormones. Your liver knows when to increase or decrease the manufacturing of cholesterol. When you take drugs to reduce the level of cholesterol in your body, you create an imbalance in your system. When you eat more cholesterol producing foods, your body makes less of it. Your body manufactures more cholesterol when you are emotionally stressed out.

Cholesterol levels are also influenced by the quality of food intake. A diet consisting of grains, beans, fruits and vegetables produces low levels of cholesterol. Diets rich in meat and high fat dairy products elevate blood cholesterol and plaque accumulates in the arteries. This type of food also has a lot of calories.

What is a Calorie?

A calorie is a unit quantity of heat. It is the amount of heat needed to raise the temperature of 1 gram of water through 1 degree C. A calorie is used to measure the energy value of foods.

What are Carbohydrates?

Carbohydrates are a large group of energy-producing organic compounds that are made of carbon, hydrogen, and oxygen such as starch, glucose, and sugar. Carbohydrates provide fuel, heat and energy for our bodily requirements.

Carbohydrates are found in grains, beans, potatoes, fruits and sugars.

What are Fats?

Fats are natural oily or greasy substances developed in our bodies. They are stored energy which is made available on demand to protect the body from changes in temperature and injuries. Some sources of fats are: milk and milk products, nuts and vegetable oils, such as soybeans, sesame, corn and sunflower.

What are Minerals?

Minerals are crystalline structures of natural inorganic substances. They are found in the earth as mineral salts, and are taken up by plants from the soil.

Minerals are involved in the chemical reactions of the body. It is very important to have a sufficient amount of minerals to prevent disease. The most important minerals are iron, calcium, iodine, sodium, potassium, phosphorus and magnesium. Some sources of minerals are fresh and dried fruits, beans, green vegetables, breads, nuts, milk and cheese.

What are Vitamins?

The word vitamin comes from the Latin word "vita", which means life, and "amine", which means amino acid. Vitamins are organic compounds, necessary for normal function and development of the body. They are required in small quantities in the diet, because they cannot be made by the body.

Deficiency or excess of vitamins is dangerous, for it may lead to different diseases. Vitamins A, B, C, D and E are essential in a number of bodily functions. For example:

Vitamin A - contributes to good eye sight, healthy skin and hair. Lack of vitamin A causes night-blindness, peeling nails, dry skin. Some sources of vitamin A are carrots, spinach, sweet potatoes, broccoli, fresh apricots and butter.

The vitamin B group - contributes to the health of every cell of the body. It is very important for normal function and maintenance of the body. Lack of vitamin B causes depression, instability and bad breath. Some sources of the vitamin B group are nuts, milk, sprouts, green vegetables, rice and whole grains.

Vitamin C (ascorbic acid) - contributes to the formation of the connective tissues which holds the cells together. Vitamin C detoxifies the blood, helps in the absorption of iron and other nutrients and also, relieves stress. Lack of vitamin C causes rapid aging, loss of teeth and fragile bones. Some sources of vitamin C are fresh fruits and vegetables, especially broccoli, green peppers, oranges and lemons.

Vitamin D (calciferol) - contributes to the absorption of calcium and phosphorus. Lack of vitamin D causes bone, tooth and gum diseases. The sources of vitamin D are milk, butter and ultraviolet rays from the sun.

Vitamin E - helps in blood circulation and preserving oxygen by the body. Lack of vitamin E causes weak muscles, heart problems and blood clots. Some sources of vitamin E are soybean oil, butter, beans and sweet potatoes.

What to Eat to Create a New You?

Your New Lifestyle Foods should contain grains, beans, vegetables, fruits, low fat milk products, nuts, herbs and spices. These foods are composed of all the necessary ingredients to attain longevity, and help create a happy and healthy You.

Let's begin our journey to an exciting and mysterious world: the world of spices. Unfortunately, the misconception that spices are hot has kept people away from freely using them in their cooking and deprived many from acquiring a balanced and healthy life.

In the next chapter you will learn why the great mariners of the world were looking for India. No, not for gold!

CHAPTER 2

THE MYSTIQUE OF SPICE

Why Were Columbus And The Rest Of The European Mariners Looking For India, And What Had Their Search To Do With Food?

"If my countryman had had
the Indian's knowledge of spices,
I would have conquered the whole world"

Baber The Great
Founder of the Mogul Empire

It is a misconception that all spices are hot and burn the tongue and stomach. This certainly is not the case with spices such as cinnamon, saffron, cumin, just to name a few. Only some members of the pepper family have that chilli-hot, spicy effect.

The importance of spice has been recognized from ancient times for its medicinal, preservative and seasoning properties. Vast sums of money were invested by powerful European monarchs of the day to find alternative sea routes to India to trade for spices. Why?

In the days when there was no refrigeration, spice was prized for its usefulness as a preservative as well as for its ability to enhance the nourishing power and taste of food. Since imported spice was scarce and as costly as gold, silver, coral and precious stones it was not affordable by the general public. Even to this day the Dutch have a saying: "It is as costly as pepper". All of the above contributed to the mystique of spice.

Now, of course, we cross continents in a matter of hours with the result that the price of Indian spice is reasonable and affordable. Its availability and the increasing awareness of the medicinal as well as the exotic qualities of spices and herbs has motivated a large number of people in Europe and America to use spice in their cooking.

What is the secret of spicing food? The magic of spicing is in the blending. It is called "Masala". Mastering the art of cooking is in knowing how to blend the different spices. The intent of this book is to make you a master in no time. You will have the key to not only cooking mouth watering dishes, but also the key to perfect health.

The third step in Romancing The Stove is to open up your mind to the world of spice, take away the prejudices of the past, and enter into the adventure of new ways of cooking and eating.

Spice Up Your Life

Most spices do not set fire to your insides. Only the hot peppers of the spice world have such an effect, and even then it depends on how much is encountered at any one time and in what strength.

We are so used to cinnamon toast, ginger bread and cumin bagels that we tend to forget that ginger, cinnamon, cumin, as well as cloves, coriander and fennel are the great exotic spices. They are medicine as well. They enhance the power of food. Learn more about them. Spice up your life and continue to enjoy living.

Next time you hear: "I cannot eat spicy food", just remember they are talking only about some hot peppers and not the exotic spices. While not everyone may like hot spices, most people enjoy the flavour of spicy food. Spice is medicine. It is a catalyst for power.

Even in our day-to-day language we say: "Spice up your life". It doesn't necessarily mean create a burning sensation.

Spice up your life and eat as much as you want!

Live a happy, healthy and beautiful life!

And above all - Eat great, tasty, delicious food!

When through practice you become familiar with the recipes contained in this book, you will find that you really begin to look forward to your meals. Eating will no longer be routine, but a celebration of the charm of life. Your taste buds and your entire body will become alert and alive: a veritable shrine for your soul.

THE NEW WAY

"Let Your Food Be Your Medicine.
Let Your Medicine Be Your Food"

Hippocrates

"If you don't get lost, you cannot find new places.
New places are new ways."

Sri Tulshi

Let me share some of my personal experiences with you. Like many people, I suffered from severe migraine headaches, indigestion, heartburn, abnormal blood pressure and acne. I didn't know what to do... I was going from one specialist to another and tried this and that diet... nothing helped.

My good fortune finally brought me to a great teacher, who introduced me to the ancient philosophy of the Vedas and the Ayurvedic system of food preparation and eating. The results were astonishing!

I learned that every herb, every grain, every spice is not only food but medicine. By combining certain spices and herbs my system was cleansed of toxins. By eating a few slices of fresh ginger combined with breathing and stretching exercises my headaches disappeared. By taking one teaspoon of Chyawanprash twice a day (Chyawanprash is an Ayurvedic herbal preparation which is available in most East Indian Grocery stores), I helped my body resist infections that led to coughs and colds; brought benefits to my nervous system; soothed my digestion; contributed to my general health and slowed down my aging process.

A turning point in my life occurred when I acquired my own supply of natural spices, herbs and dried fruits and put them in glass jars in my kitchen cupboard. By using these ingredients mixed and combined according to the Ayurvedic system I experienced a New Birth!

My health improved dramatically after eating the most exciting foods I have ever eaten in my entire life. And believe you me, I have been to some of the best restaurants around the world, from Paris to Hong Kong and Taipei!

You too can empower your life, improve your health, have fun and enjoy the most sumptuous food. Let me show you the way.

The fourth step of Romancing The Stove is to discover the secret of using spices to enhance the taste of your food, and the effect spices have on the body and mind.

THE HIDDEN POWER OF HERBS AND SPICES

The Secret
Of Enhancing The Taste Of Your Food And
The Effects Of Spice On The Body And Mind -
According To The Ancient Science of India,
Ayurveda - "The Science of Life"

(Pre Hippocrates and Paracelsus)

Below is a list of spices we will be using throughout Romancing The Stove. We also give some Ayurvedic attributes to each of these spices. Next to the English names, we include in brackets the Hindi name of the same spice as this may be of help if you go shopping in an Indian grocery store.

ASAFOETIDA (Hing) - root of the parsley family plant, dried and ground, has strong aroma and great medicinal value.

Effects On The Body:

Stimulant, digestive, aphrodisiac, antiseptic. A perfect cleanser after eating meats, fish and junk foods. Helps to get rid of stagnated foods, relieves gas, colic pain, constipation. Externally used as a paste for arthritic and abdominal pain.

Effects On The Mind:

Tamasic: grounding, down to Earth, relaxing.

In Cooking:

It can replace onion and garlic. Good with ginger and cardamom to reduce gas. Use sparingly. Store in tight container.

WILD CELERY SEEDS (Ajwan) - small green seeds.

Effects On The Body:

Stimulant, antispasmodic, energizing. An excellent help for digestion, kidney function, removing intestinal gas and spasms, sinus congestion and breathing.

Effects On The Mind:

Rajasic: a good nerve stimulant. A vitalizer for the throat chakra. Improves speech and promotes clear communications and creativity.

In Cooking:

Has strong aroma, sprinkle sparingly on breads, noodles, potatoes, beans.

BASIL (Tulshi) - a sun loving aromatic herb. A very popular plant of India.

Effects On The Body:

Antibacterial and antiseptic. Helps to remove congestion, headaches, abdominal pains, colds.

Effects On The Mind:

Sattvic: opens the flow of energy, strengthening and purifying the aura. It gives clarity to the mind, increases memory. It is good to keep a basil plant in the home, as an air purifier. Wearing string beads made out of Tulshi stems balances energy.

In Cooking:

It is best to use it fresh. Dried basil leaves loose their fragrance. Fresh basil juice with honey helps to clear the mind and strengthen the nerves.

BLACK PEPPER (Gol Marich) - whole peppercorns, or lightly roasted and ground.

Effects On The Body:

A very powerful digestive, removes toxins from the colon, cleanses stagnated foods, helps in constipation, obesity and colds.

Effects On The Mind:

Rajasic: adds excitement, compassion and strength.

In Cooking:

Used in rice, vegetables, lentils; very good with cold raw vegetables (cucumbers and salads). Better if roasted before use.

CARDAMOM SEEDS (Elaichi) - small fruit of a plant with very aromatic black seeds. The most popular spice of India.

Effects On The Body:

Digestive stimulant, tonic for the heart, helps to strengthen the nervous and blood circulation systems.

Effects On The Mind:

Sattvic: soothing, opens the flow of energy to the body, balancing the body and mind. Enhances spiritual work and meditation.

In Cooking:

Used in making sweets and drinks, spiced teas. Excellent mouth freshener. Used in rice, lentils and vegetable dishes to increase digestion. For best flavour use cardamom in green pods.

CAYENNE PEPPER (Marichi-phalam) - also called Chilli pepper, the fruit of the sun. Varies in length and heat potency (shorter chillies are usually hotter then longer ones). Enhances the taste and aromas of many other herbs. It is stronger than black pepper.

Effects On The Body:

Very effective in burning toxins from the colon. Helps in indigestion, poor absorption, abdominal distention, worms, sinus congestion, poor circulation. Strengthens the heart. If over used can aggravate the body.

Effects On The Mind:

Rajasic: adds excitement, creates heat in the body, adds strength. It can disturb the mind if overused.

In Cooking:

We use them whole. This spice makes your food really hot. If you don't like hot food, eliminate chillies from your recipes. But if you want to benefit from the medicinal value of cayenne peppers, fry them quickly in hot ghee or oil and remove them before adding the liquid: water or yogurt. Remember the hottest part of cayenne pepper is in the seeds. Do not crush the chillies. Use them whole.

CINNAMON (Dalchini) - bark of the cinnamon tree. Used both as small sticks and as ground cinnamon.

Effects On The Body:

A very effective help for the circulation, pain reliever for toothache and muscle tension. Strengthens the heart and warms the body.

Effects On The Mind:

Sattvic: warms and soothes the body and mind. Balances the flow of energy, enhances meditation and spiritual activities.

In Cooking:

Used in sauces, rice dishes, vegetables. Good in beverages. Together with cardamom and bay leaves helps promote digestion and absorption of other foods. Remove cinnamon stick before serving food.

CLOVES (Lavanga) - dried flower buds from tropical evergreen trees of the myrtle family.

Effects On The Body:

Very effective stimulant for the lungs and stomach, helps with colds, coughs, toothaches, indigestion. Aphrodisiac, helps with impotence and low blood pressure.

Effects On The Mind:

Rajasic: adds excitement, passion, strength. Inspires and energizes. But if over used, can create irritation.

In Cooking:

An excellent mouth freshener. Good in beverages, rice and dal. Remove cloves before serving food.

CORIANDER (Dhaniya) - Chinese parsley, also called Cilantro. Used as a fresh herb, or as seeds.

Effects On The Body:

Very effective herb for digestion and absorption of other herbs and foods. Helps to dissolve blockages, relieve spasms, gas and intestinal pains. The fresh juice of coriander leaves helps in allergies, itches and skin rashes. Fresh coriander is a good source of protein and vitamin C.

Effects On The Mind:

Sattvic: cooling, soothing, opens the flow of energy to the body, uplifting to the spirit, balancing to body and mind.

In Cooking:

To have the best effect from fresh coriander leaves, add them just before serving. To have the best result from coriander seeds, roast them first then grind. Excellent with rice, vegetables, soups, salads, beverages.

CUMIN SEEDS (Jeera) - Small, sweet seeds. Could be light or dark in colour.

Effects On The Body:

Helps to increase digestion, absorption and assimilation of other herbs and foods. Helps to remove gas and indigestion. Also a rejuvenative.

Effects On The Mind:

Sattvic: cooling, soothing, rejuvenating and healing for the nervous system. Helps in balancing the solar plexus chakra.

In Cooking:

We use whole cumin seeds daily. Dry roasted and ground cumin seeds are good with rice, dal, vegetables, yogurt dishes, relishes, snacks and salads.

FENNEL SEEDS (Souf) - Larger and greener than cumin seeds with anise-like flavour. It is sometimes called: "Old ladies' chewing tobacco", or "Sweet cumin".

Effects On The Body:

Great helper for cleaning internal organs and removing toxins. Digestive, stimulant, rejuvenative. Good for nursing mothers to increase flow of milk.

Effects On The Mind:

Sattvic: calming and soothing for the nerves.

In Cooking:

Dry roasted it is good as a mouth freshener. They are part of the Bengal five-spice mixture called Panch Phoron, used often in cooking vegetables, lentils, soups, pickles, snacks. Can be substituted by anise seeds.

FENUGREEK (Methi) - fresh green herb or yellow seeds.

Effects On The Body:

Very good rejuvenative, strengthens the reproductive, nervous and respiratory systems. Good for hair growth. Helps digestion, liver disorders and increases semen. Good for woman after child birth to increase milk flow and strengthen the body.

Effects On The Mind:

Rajasic: adds excitement and strength, uplifts and stimulates body and mind.

In Cooking:

As a tonic can be taken daily (1 tsp. of powder heated in one cup of milk). Good in soups, vegetables and tonic drinks.

GINGER (Adrak) - use as a fresh root or powder.

Effects On The Body:

Very good for indigestion. Relieves gas and cramps in the abdomen. Offers help for arthritis and headaches. Ginger tea is an aid for colds and stomach problems. A tonic for the heart. Often called The Universal Medicine.

Effects On The Mind:

Sattvic: balances the flow of energy. Good for people who meditate and do spiritual work.

In Cooking:

We use it daily in soups, vegetable dishes, milk beverages and teas.

MINT (Pudina) - fresh green aromatic leaves.

Effects On The Body:

Helps as a digestive. A nervine, respiratory, circulatory stimulant. Also helps with colds, sore throats, headaches, laryngitis, nausea and vomiting.

Effects On The Mind:

Sattvic: cooling and soothing effect on the body and mind. Relieves tension and congestion.

In Cooking:

Best when used fresh in teas and chutney's.

MUSTARD SEEDS (Rai) - small, round, black or yellow seeds (our preference is black seeds).

Effects On The Body:

Helps as stimulant and digestive, increases internal heat and circulation, destroys accumulation of toxins, enhances assimilation of food.

Effects On The Mind:

Rajasic: stimulates the senses, creates excitement, increases vitality.

In Cooking:

Excellent in cooking green vegetables, potatoes, rice and dal. Often used together with other stimulant herbs and spices, like cayenne pepper, black pepper, cinnamon, cloves, fennel, fenugreek, asafoetida, ginger, onion seeds.

TURMERIC (Haldi) - fresh as an orange-yellow root of the ginger family, or as dry powder.

Effects On The Body:

Natural antibiotic, antibacterial, stimulant and purifier of the blood. A cleanser of all tissues of the body. Helps in poor circulation, indigestion, arthritis, anaemia, cuts and bruises. Also helps to digest protein from other foods.

Effects On The Mind:

Sattvic: purifies all chakras. Balances mind, body and spirit, creating harmony and peace.

In Cooking:

Excellent in soups, vegetables, beverages, rice dishes and lentils.

The next step in Romancing The Stove is to find the secret path to longevity through preforming the basic rules in the celebration of eating.

CHAPTER 3

A CELEBRATION OF EATING

The Seven Golden Rules - A Path To Longevity

Eating is an offering to the body. The senses feel gratified when we offer wholesome and tasteful food to this place (body) we call home.

We suggest an ancient ritual, a Vedic system of eating. Legend has it that it is a path to longevity. Here are the basic requirements for performing the celebration of eating:

1. **The place** where you eat should be quiet and peaceful. You should not have any disturbing or unpleasant conversations during your meal. You should not discuss any business or read a newspaper or book.

2. **The best time** of the day for your main meal is at midday when digestion is the highest. Eat three times per day. Breakfast and dinner should be light.

3. **The interval** of six hours has to be maintained between meals. You have to give your stomach enough time for digestion.

4. **The sequence** in which food should be eaten is important. The food you eat first should be sweeter in taste, such as grains and legumes. These foods contain the body building materials: proteins and amino acids. They should fill up one third of your stomach.

Next in order should be sour and salty foods, such as cooked vegetables, soups, yogurt and salads. They increase digestion and fill up the next third of the stomach.

Salads should not be eaten at the beginning of the meal, for they create gas and constipation.

5. **At the end** of the meal you should take half a cup of fresh yogurt mixed with half a cup of water (buttermilk-lassi) to stimulate digestion, avoid gas and maintain a proper acid-alkaline balance in the stomach.

For proper digestion: the first third of your stomach should be filled with solid foods, the second third with water or more liquid based foods and finally, the third part of your stomach should be left empty.

6. **After the meal** do not drink for one hour. Rest for about ten minutes. Let the fire of digestion do its work.

About one hour later to quench your thirst you can drink anything you like. Try our empowering hot teas and cold drinks.

7. **State of mind** during the meal has to be peaceful. Correct eating will create a happy human being, balanced and satisfied with life. If the body feels heavy and tired, if the mind becomes numb and dull, it means that the yoga of eating did not take place. The process of eating was not properly accomplished.

Balance is the key. Moderation in eating and sleeping will prolong your life. Excessive and deficient eating and sleeping will disturb the balance in your system and develop stress, pain and disease.

The seven Golden Rules,
combined with the right mix of dishes in this program can
create harmony of body and mind, resulting in a balanced life.

Part two of this book takes you to the next step and shows you how to get ready before you start Romancing The Stove.

PART TWO

OVERTURE TO THE CREATION

CHAPTER 4

OPENING NOTES

Before You Start Romancing The Stove
You Must Get Ready

Every home has its unique character which reflects the taste and living style of its residents. Equally distinctive is the way our sense of smell is affected by the owners preferences in cooking, whether they smoke or not, or burn incense, use perfumes or any number of other factors. Some homes can be fragrant and inviting while others are less so.

It is the same with food preparation. Ten people could cook the same dish, using the same recipes from the same cook book and yet the taste and aroma would be somewhat different in each case.

Why? Because it depends on how the recipes were followed, on the freshness of the herbs, spices and the other ingredients, on the amount of time the spices were sizzled or roasted and on the individual use of the Phoron technique (see page 45).

Therefore, let's agree to use the freshest and the most wholesome looking ingredients that we can find for our food preparation - but allow yourself to be free, have fun and add or delete ingredients according to your taste.

Most of us would probably have no objections to the observation that home cooking, properly prepared with loving care and made with natural ingredients is far superior to commercially made or restaurant fare. It is so enjoyable to make your own yogurt, clarified butter, cheese and chutney... try it, see for yourself.

Enter the romance and experience the creation!

The Milky Way To Longevity, Memory and Intelligence

Our basic recipes for home-made milk products include clarified butter (ghee), fresh cheese (paneer), yogurt (dahi) and buttermilk (lassi)

Why did we include milk and milk products in the basic recipes? Because they must be a part of our daily sustenance and for their divine qualities. Milk was praised in the ancient Vedic scriptures for its high concentration of the nutrients necessary for health. Yogis rely on milk for its calming, rejuvenating, life- giving and healing properties.

My suggestion is to use 2% milk as it has more substance and is better tasting than skim milk. Remember, your body needs some fat in the diet to assist in the absorption of calcium and other organic processes. For those who are lactose intolerant, milk can be purchased in which lactose has been modified for better digestion. In that same regard, according to Ayurvedic practice, boiling milk before its use not only disposes of unwanted bacteria but also improves its digestibility.

Let us think of milk as a naturally occurring miraculous food that can assist us in living a full and rich life. Now we want to find out more about how to prepare milk for its various products and how to combine it with other foods.

Seven Secrets For Getting The Best Results
When Using Dairy

1. Milk should be taken daily and in moderation (adults: about two cups; children: about three cups; nursing mothers: about six cups). It helps to remove toxins from the system and strengthen the body.

2. Milk is an ideal culture for the growth of bacteria. It should be boiled before it is used. As has been said previously, boiling assists in the digestion of milk and in controlling unwanted bacteria.

3. Milk should not be taken cold and with other foods because it is harder to digest cold milk. We recommend drinking milk hot with added spices (see our recipes).

4. Yogurt is a good accompaniment to other foods, but not by itself. It benefits the reproductive system and the blood, and improves the population of beneficial microbes in the intestine.

5. Buttermilk is best for digestion. It is good to take it daily, 1/2 cup after the main meal. It helps to remove toxins and balance the cholesterol level in the body system.

6. Butter gives vitality to the body, but it should be taken in moderation, for it develops fat. It helps in coughs, intestinal disorders, hemorrhoid and other diseases.

7. Clarified butter (ghee) is called "Liquid Gold". It is good for any age. Ghee helps to increase longevity and memory. It is very good for chest problems, stomach problems, skin problems; and it also benefits the reproduction system. Preparation is the key. To prepare home made milk products see our recipes: The Foundation Of Romance, The Shape Of Tenderness, The Romantic's Delight and The Milk Of Human Kindness.

The Foundation Of Romance -
Clarified Butter (Ghee)

Experience The Touch Of Class,
The Taste Of Liquid Gold

Clarified butter, called Ghee, is the very essence of butter. It takes about 4 hours of slow cooking to purify 4 pounds of butter. Purify or clarify means to fully evaporate the water and to separate the milk solids from the butter.

People call it Liquid Gold for its gorgeous golden colour. Besides the colour it has an exquisite flavour, a warm, inviting aroma and high medicinal values. It is an ideal medium for cooking and it will add a wonderful flavour to your dishes. Ghee will not burn and smoke easily because all the impurities have been removed from it.

According to Ayurvedic medicine, Ghee, in moderation, will not increase the cholesterol level in your blood; it will not clog your liver but strengthen it; it will feed your brain, nerve and reproductive systems; it will empower your digestive system; it will strengthen your body and mind; it will help to increase your memory and intelligence and add to your longevity. Ghee is perfect for the young and old. Try it, you will love it!

Here is how to create The Foundation Of Romance:

Use 4 lbs. of unsalted butter

Use a large heavy pot

1. Bring butter to boil.
2. Lower heat and let it simmer for about 4 hours, or till golden.
3. Remove from stove.
4. Strain it through cheese cloth.
5. Ghee does not need refrigeration.

***Warning: Do not overcook. It will spoil the flavour and become dark.

The Shape Of Tenderness -
Home Made Yogurt (Dahi)

You can include yogurt's gentle presence in almost every meal. Sages seldom eat yogurt by itself, but always with other foods. Yogurt is usually served plain and unsweetened along with the meal.

Yogurt has great healing power. It has natural antibiotic qualities. It benefits the reproductive system and the blood. It helps to digest food. It has important vitamins and minerals, proteins and enzymes. It is downright tasty. Here is how to make yogurt:

3 litres warm milk

3 tbsp. plain yogurt (to be used as culture)

1. Bring milk to boil.
2. Remove from heat and let it cool.
3. Place 3 tbsp. of previously made yogurt, as a culture, in a glass or ceramic pot in which you plan to make fresh yogurt.
4. Add warm milk, stir and leave in a warm place overnight.
5. After the yogurt is made it must be kept in the refrigerator.
6. Serve unsweetened with meals.

The Milk Of Human Kindness -
Home Made Buttermilk (Lassi)

Buttermilk is home-made yogurt diluted with an equal amount of water and blended in a mixer. According to Ayurveda, 1/2 a glass of buttermilk should be taken daily after the main meal. You can make it sweet, or salty depending on your preference. It increases the digestive power, helps to remove gas, toxins and extra fat from the system. It helps to control the cholesterol level, helps to heal ulcers, liver problems and colic. Here is how to prepare The Milk Of Human Kindness:

Preparation time: 2 minutes.
Serves 4.

1 cup yogurt
1 cup water
1/2 tsp. sea salt (or raw sugar)
1/2 tsp. fresh ginger root (grated)
1/4 tsp. roasted and ground coriander seeds
1/4 tsp. roasted and ground cumin seeds

1. Blend all ingredients together and serve right away.

Romantic's Delight -
Fresh Home Made Cheese (Paneer)

Paneer is something that every one should try. It is the most delicious and healthiest cheese ever. No preservatives and no chemicals are added. It is pure and powerful. We love it.

Paneer is warm, tender and sweet when it is just made. It can be eaten plain or with raw honey, maple syrup or salt and pepper. It can be added to vegetable dishes, rice or soups and it can be used for cooking different dishes and sweets after it has been pressed overnight to remove excess moisture.

Preparation of paneer takes about 20 minutes, as long as it takes to boil the milk. From 4 litres of milk you can make about 500 grams of unpressed cheese or about 400 grams of pressed cheese.

Try it. You will very quickly feel the flow of energy and power through your body. It is easy. It is fun. Here is how to make fresh Paneer:

4 litres of milk

2 fresh limes/lemons

1. Bring milk to boil.
2. Remove from heat and squeeze lime/lemon juice into the boiled milk.
3. Stir and see how the curds of paneer separate from the greenish whey.
4. Strain to separate the cheese from the whey using some cheesecloth.
5. Serve warm with raw honey, maple syrup, or salt and pepper.

*** Note: For making cheese dishes, place cheesecloth with cheese between two large plates. Put something heavy on top, and let it stay under the pressure overnight, or till firm.

CHAPTER 5

FLAVOURS TRANSCENDENT

Tamarind - The Legend

Tamarind is an exotic fruit. Legend says that saplings of this tree were brought from Atlantis to India where the Atlanteans settled after Atlantis submerged in the Atlantic ocean.

Its taste is unique. It transcends the limitations of words to describe the taste of tamarind. You have to taste it to know what it is like.

The Arabs, who brought tamarind back from India after their conquests, called it "Tamar Hindi" which means "Indian date". The epitome of Arab fruits is the date which shades the oasis and exorcises the hunger of weary desert travellers. By naming tamarind "Indian date", they paid the highest respect to this fruit and by including it in their cooking they extended that respect.

Tamarind has a mystical taste. It is neither sour nor sweet; it transcends both. Craving for a touch of tamarind sauce can make your mouth flood with juices. It can make a simple slice of potato or boiled chic peas into a gourmet dish. The base of the taste is tart with a hint of bitter and a touch of sweet. The taste buds are enlivened with overtures of sweet and sour.

All sensations of taste are in this healing fruit. Its juices help digestion. It is like an escort of entrees. That is why all Indian food is served with tamarind sauce and often in combination with mint.

Try it. It is truly a divine experience when you put tamarind sauce on the tip of your tongue - your whole body will vibrate and eating will become rapturous.

The Stimulant - Tamarind Sauce (Imli)

Add an exotic touch to your meals
Feel warm and light, cleansed and joyful

Use tamarind pulp in preference to whole pressed tamarind. It is available in Indian grocery stores. Tamarind sauce is a great stimulant. To add more sweetness and an exotic taste, mix it with dates.

Here is how to make The Stimulant:

1 cup tamarind pulp

1/2 cup dried dates

2 cups boiling water

1/4 tsp. sea salt, or to taste

1/4 tsp. red chilli powder, or to taste

1. Pour boiling water over tamarind and dates and soak over night.
2. Strain through strainer to extract all of the juice, then throw the pulp away.
3. Add salt and chilli powder.
4. Mix all ingredients together.
5. Fill up jars with caps and keep refrigerated (good for about one week).

Serve with any lunch or dinner.

The Heart Warming Blend Of Spices;
Not Hot At All - Garam Masala

This warming mixture has a beautiful and strong aroma
It is also a great stimulant for digestion

Garam masala is a blend of aromatic spices which are usually used at the end of cooking to intensify the aroma and flavour.

Garam means warming-hot, but not chilli-hot; and masala means a mixture of spices. This warming blend not only enhances the joy of eating but also stimulates digestion.

Garam masala is often used in yogurt dishes, lentil soups and vegetables. The proportions and ingredients may be changed to suit individual taste. Here is how to make Garam Masala:

4 cinnamon sticks, 3 inches long

4 tbsp. cumin seeds

2 tbsp. black peppercorns (optional)

2 tbsp. cloves

1 nutmeg

2 tbsp. cardamom seeds

4 tbsp. coriander seeds

1. Heat the frying pan over medium heat.
2. Put all ingredients in the frying pan, stir and dry roast till a shade darker.
3. Cool and grind.
4. Cover tightly and store until required.

*** Warning: Do not make a large portion of this blend for it loses freshness with time. Keep it away from heat and dampness in a covered jar.

The Secret Treasures Of Your Pantry

Amaze Your Family And Friends
With Flavours Transcendent

Create sensational flavour by adding roasted and freshly ground coriander seeds and cumin seeds to your food before serving your meal, or at the very end of cooking. Feel the exciting aromas. Enjoy the variety and richness of flavours. Discover the mysterious, exotic taste hidden in familiar spices.

Roasted And Ground Coriander Seeds

5 tbsp. whole coriander seeds

Heavy frying pan

Coffee grinder

1.   Heat frying pan over medium heat.
2.   Add coriander seeds, stir and dry roast them till brown.
3.   Cool, grind and store in covered jar until required.

Roasted And Ground Cumin Seeds

5 tbsp. whole cumin seeds

Heavy frying pan

Coffee grinder

Use the same technique as above.

The Sages Quintessence -
A Unique Mingling Of Spices - Panch Phoron

An Equal Mixture Of Five Whole (Not Ground) Spices

This mixture of spices brings out the subtle taste of different foods and motivates the taste buds to go into rapture. It is very popular in Bengal.

Panch Phoron is a Bengali name which means five spices. Panch means five and Phoron means spicing up or adding (see page 45). This unique combination of spices can make a simple vegetarian dish or lentil soup into a meal for a connoisseur.

5 tbsp. black mustard seeds

5 tbsp. cumin seeds

5 tbsp. onion seeds (kalonji)*

5 tbsp. fennel seeds

5 tbsp. fenugreek seeds

1. Mix all ingredients together.
2. Store in a tightly covered jar and use according to our recipes.
3. Good for a long time if kept away from heat and dampness.

* Kalonji - Black onion seeds can be found in Indian grocery stores.

The Heart Of Cooking - The Phoron Technique

Adding spice during the process of cooking is called Phoron. The secret of extracting the real flavour of vegetables and grains is in the following:

a) The spice you add, ground or whole.

b) At what stage of the cooking you add these spices.

c) How long the spices must be cooked or sizzled.

d) The sequence in which the spices are mixed.

e) Finally, the quantity of spices added to each dish.

At first glance it may appear to be an elaborate process, but when you get down to doing it you will find it as simple as one, two, three. In each recipe we have given you the quantity of spices, the timing and the sequence of adding the spices. Here is how we do it:

1. In a small pot, heat some ghee and add dried spices or herbs, for example: dried chilli, bay leaves and sizzle till brown.

2. Add whole dried seeds according to the recipe, for example: cumin, fenugreek, fennel, kalonji, black mustard seeds and sizzle until they pop.

3. Add powdered, grated, or ground spices according to the recipe, for example: turmeric, ginger and asafoetida.

4. Add vegetables, rice, or grains and stir fry for a few minutes until they absorb the aroma and medicinal values of the spices.

5. Add liquids according to the recipe for example: water, yogurt, or soup.

PART THREE

CREATING WEALTH

CHAPTER 6

HEALTH IS WEALTH

Creating Your Own Wealth

Driven by necessity and the desire to get ahead, men and women work such long hours that they don't have enough time to eat properly. That is why the fast food industry is a multi-billion dollar business.

I recently suggested to a very successful doctor who is a naturopath, to send a thank you note to all the major fast food chains for his increase in clientele.

The axiom "Health is Wealth" needs no explanation. What will you do with your millions, if your body is sick? If you are sick you are very poor indeed, regardless of how much money you have.

Health is wealth. A healthy body is a reflection of a healthy mind. And a healthy body and mind are the basis for a life of peace and joy.

Now you have come to the point when you are ready to take the final step to create your wealth, to master the art of cooking and eating, to enhance your romance and live a healthy, fulfilling life. Before we start, let us summarize all the steps of the Romancing The Stove program:

*** In the first step you got acquainted with eating the natural way in order to maintain a healthy body and mind.

*** In the second step you found out more about the food you eat so that you could create more balance and harmony in your life.

*** In the third step you opened up your mind to the mystique of spices, to spice up your life and invigorate your body. You also realized, that spice is not hot peppers only.

*** In the fourth step you found out the secrets of using spices to enhance the taste of your food, and the effects of spices on your body and mind.

*** In the fifth step you found the secret path to longevity through performing the basic rules in the celebration of eating to create a healthy body. You learned that a healthy body, in turn, will provide you with the right conditions for a happy mind and a romantic spirit.

*** In the sixth step you made yourself ready for Romancing The Stove.

*** In the final, and the seventh step you will experience what only a healthy body, a happy mind and a romantic spirit can bring you. Since health is wealth, you will also experience the thrill of creating your own wealth.

Since the quality and kind of food we eat is the basis of a healthy or an unhealthy body we may conclude that health food can also be called wealth food.

Generally, most people's perception of health food is that it is tasteless, insipid, and a torture for the palate. But it does not have to be so if you let Romancing The Stove show you the way.

The author has gone through the horrors of insipid, tasteless food in her struggle to attain emotional and physical health. The result of this excruciatingly painful experience and subsequent events finally led her to the discovery of these luscious mouthwatering dishes. Now she shares this acquired wealth with you. So, get ready and enjoy this wealth food.

CHAPTER 7

EXOTIC DISHES

A Grandmother Called Saroju
Whom I Have Never Met

The exotic dishes compiled in this chapter originated in a very cosy and affectionate kitchen of my teacher's grandmother who had imparted to him the formula for the joyous way to master the cooking of wealth food and the wisdom behind it.

She had raised eleven very healthy children from that kitchen. They loved to eat and they grew to be big boys and girls. They became world famous movie makers, lawyers and entrepreneurs. They were seldom, if ever sick, and they ate to their heart's content.

When my teacher talked to me about this way of cooking he did so in a loving voice saying that this is how his grandmother would do it. He told me many stories about her.

I have never met my teacher's grandmother, but I feel I have known her all my life. It is as if I was sitting in her kitchen, she was doing the cooking and giving me her very personal instructions. In essence she has a hand in writing Romancing The Stove.

Now let us enter her famous kitchen...

The Exotica De Bengal -
Spiced Potato And Cabbage

Enjoy the exotic taste of Bengal cooking. This taste transcends description. But more than that, it is a tonic to strengthen the liver and purify the blood. It is a freshener for the body and a joy for the taste buds.

Preparation time: 40 minutes
Serves 4-6

2 tbsp. clarified butter (ghee)
2 dried red chilli (optional)
2 bay leaves
4 medium potatoes (cubed)
1 small cabbage (washed, and minced)
1 tsp. sea salt
1/2 tsp. ground roasted cumin
1/2 tsp. ground roasted coriander
1/2 tsp. asafoetida
2 tbsp. fresh ginger root (grated)
1/2 tsp. turmeric
1 cup water
2 tbsp. coriander leaves (finely chopped)

1. Heat ghee, add red chilli, bay leaves and sizzle till brown.
2. Add potatoes and fry till golden, about 10 minutes.
3. Add cabbage and the rest of ingredients.
4. Mix all the spices, and stir fry for 10 minutes.
5. Add water, cover and lower the heat.
6. Cook for 20 more minutes, or till vegetables are ready.
7. Garnish with fresh coriander leaves. Serve hot.

The Ultimate Tango -
Cottage Cheese With Peas

Cheese and peas is a delicacy traditionally called Mater Paneer. Mater means peas and Paneer means home made cottage cheese. The name does not give justice to this delicacy. It is a sumptuous dish with a very tender aroma and flavour. It is perfect with hot plain rice or whole wheat unleavened bread to make a complete meal.

Preparation time: 20 minutes.

Serves 4-6.

(Make paneer a day before cooking and leave it under pressure until it becomes solid).

2 tbsp. ghee

1 tsp. cumin seeds

4 medium tomatoes (chopped)

1 tbsp. fresh ginger root (grated)

1/2 tsp. turmeric

1/4 chilli powder

1/2 tsp. ground coriander

1 tsp. sea salt, or to taste

1 tsp. raw sugar (jaggery)

2 cups peas

1 cup water

1 cup yogurt

1 fresh green chilli (optional)

2 cups paneer (cut into cubes)

2 tbsp. fresh coriander leaves (chopped)

1. Heat ghee, add chilli, cumin and sizzle for 30 seconds.
2. Add tomatoes, peas, the rest of the spices and mix well.
3. Mix water and yogurt in a separate bowl.
4. Add this mixture and bring to a boil.
5. Cover, lower heat and cook for 15 minutes.
6. Add panner and simmer for 5 more minutes.
7. Garnish with fresh coriander leaves. Serve hot with rice.

The Paradoxical Waltz -
Potatoes With White Radish

The paradoxical waltz of two earthy vegetables. They both grow below the ground. Extract the best out of both of them. A taste to remember. Don't even try to describe it. It invigorates the body and awakens the senses - get ready to compose a poem in the midst of eating.

Preparation time: 20 minutes.
Serves 4-6.

2 tbsp. ghee
1 dried red chilli (optional)
2 bay leaves
1/2 tsp. kalonji (onion seeds)
1/2 tsp. mustard seeds
4 medium potatoes (peeled and cubed)
1 medium white radish (peeled and cubed)
1/2 tsp. asafoetida
1/2 tsp. turmeric
1 tsp. sea salt
1/2 cup water
2 tbsp. coriander leaves (chopped)

1. Heat ghee, add red chilli, bay leaves and sizzle till brown.
2. Add kalonji and mustard seeds and sizzle till they pop.
3. Add potatoes, radish, asafoetida, turmeric and sea salt.
4. Stir and fry till golden brown.
5. Add 1/2 cup of water, cover and lower the heat.
6. Cook for 10 more minutes or till vegetables are ready.
7. Garnish with coriander leaves. Serve hot over rice.

The Power House -
Spinach And Potato

The traditional name of this dish is Aloo-Saag. Aloo means potato, and Saag means green vegetable, usually spinach. Together with plain rice it makes a complete dinner.

Wrestlers and body builders, poets and musicians will find everything they need in this dish. It is a perfect blend of brains and brawn.

Preparation time: 20 minutes. Serves 4-6.

1 tbsp. ghee

1 dried red chilli (optional)

2 bay leaves

1/2 tsp. cumin seeds

1/4 tsp. anise seeds

1/2 tsp. fennel seeds

4 medium potatoes (peeled and cubed)

2 medium tomatoes (minced)

2 bunches of spinach

1/2 tsp. turmeric

1/4 tsp. asafoetida

1 tbsp. fresh ginger root (grated)

1/2 tsp. sea salt

1. Heat ghee, add chilli and bay leaves. Sizzle till brown.
2. Add cumin, anise, fennel and sizzle till they pop.
3. Add potatoes and fry till golden brown.
4. Add tomatoes, spinach, turmeric, asafoetida, ginger, sea salt.
5. Cover and let it cook for 2 minutes.
6. Lower the heat, stir well and cook for 10 more minutes.
7. Serve hot with plain rice.

The Soothing Touch -
Okra And Potato

The Soothing Touch. This name perfectly describes the softening, soothing and cooling qualities of this dish. It is good for someone who feels a bit down or has some kind of irritation in the system. It helps in sore throats and colds.

Enjoy and benefit from the cooling, comforting and soothing touch of this delicious dish.

Preparation time: 20 minutes.
Serves 4-6.

2 tbsp. ghee (1 tbsp. for potatoes, 1 tbsp. for okra)
4 potatoes (cubed)
1 cup water (1/2 for potatoes, 1/2 for okra)
1-2 dried red chilli (optional)
1/2 tsp. mustard seeds
1/2 tsp. cumin seeds
1 lb. okra (ends cut off and halved)
1 tsp. sea salt
1/2 tsp. turmeric
2 tbsp. fresh coriander leaves (chopped)

1. Heat 1 tbsp. ghee, add potatoes and fry till golden brown.
2. Add 1/2 cup water, cover, lower heat and cook till ready.
3. In a separate frying pan heat 1 tbsp. ghee, add chilli, mustard, cumin and sizzle till they pop.
4. Add okra, salt, turmeric and stir fry for 2 minutes.
5. Add 1/2 cup water, cover, lower heat and cook for 15 more minutes.
6. Add cooked potatoes to cooked okra and stir well.
7. Garnish with coriander. Serve hot with plain rice.

Venus And Mars On A Plate - Zucchini And Tomatoes

This blend of green zucchini and red tomato, combined with plain rice, will bring you great satisfaction. It will reinforce and stimulate, strengthen and awaken.

Preparation time: 20 minutes. Serves 4-6.

1 tbsp. ghee (1/2 tbsp. for potatoes, 1/2 tbsp. for zucchini)

5 medium potatoes (cubed)

1/2 cup water

1-2 dried red chilli (optional)

2 bay leaves

1 tsp. mustard seeds

1/2 tsp. cumin seeds

1/2 tsp. ajwan seeds

3 cups tomatoes (cut small pieces)

1 tsp. sea salt

1/2 tsp. turmeric

3 large zucchini (peeled and sliced)

1/2 tsp. asafoetida

1/2 tsp. roasted and ground coriander seeds

2 tsp. honey (unpasteurized)

2 tbsp. coriander leaves (chopped)

1. Heat 1/2 tbsp. ghee, add potatoes and fry till golden brown.
2. Add 1/2 cup water, cover, lower heat and cook till ready.
3. Heat 1/2 tbsp. ghee in a large heavy pot.
4. Add chilli, bay leaves and sizzle till brown.
5. Add mustard, cumin and ajwan.
6. Add tomatoes, salt, turmeric and cook for 5 minutes.
7. Add zucchini cook for 10 more minutes.
8. Add cooked potatoes, mix well all together.
9. Before serving add roasted and ground coriander seeds, honey and salt to taste and garnish with coriander leaves. Serve hot with plain rice.

Hindu Russi Bhai! Bhai! -
Not Just Another Cabbage Roll

Russian Cabbage Rolls With Indian Stuffing

A great dish for a special occasion. It does take a little more time to prepare this delicacy than the other recipes, but it is worth your effort. Your guests and your palate will be dazzled and they will remember this experience even after all other memories have faded.

Preparation time 50 minutes. Serves 4-6.

10 cabbage leaves (boiled)
3 tbsp. sunflower oil (1 tbsp. for spices, 2 tbsp. for cabbage rolls)
1 dried red chilli (optional)
3 bay leaves
1 tsp. garam masala
1 tsp. tumeric
1- 2 green chilli (optional)
1 tsp. sea salt
2 tbsp. coriander leaves (chopped)
2 cups fresh home made cheese (paneer)

1. Boil cabbage leaves for 10 minutes and drain.
2. Heat 1 tbsp. oil, add red chilli, bay leaves and sizzle till lightly brown.
3. Add garam masala (see page 42), tumeric, chopped green chilli, sea salt, coriander leaves and sizzle for a few seconds.
4. Add paneer and stir fry for 5 minutes.
5. Remove from the stove.
6. Fill up the cabbage leaves with paneer, fold and tie with string.
7. Heat 2 tbsp. of oil and fry cabbage rolls on both sides till golden brown.
8. Serve hot.

CHAPTER 8

FOOD FOR THE GODS

The Delicacies From The Temple

It is a ritual in the Himalayan temples to offer food to the gods or deities. The same food is then distributed as a prosadam, meaning offering, to the devotees and to all who come to the temple.

While this food is conducive to the health of the body, it also has other special properties and is called "Sattvic" food. Sattva is a Sanskrit word which means light, truth, intelligence and harmony; all of which make it especially suitable for those who are following a spiritual practice. It is a perfect mind-body-spirit balanced food and is a joy to eat. It's fragrance can match the fragrance of the soul. It is the healthiest food one can enjoy in this three dimensional world. The beauty of this offering is that it never leaves you feeling sluggish. This food will give you the energy to withstand ecstasy and overcome all obstacles on your spiritual journey.

Come, let's invoke the mighty Himalayas and the Masters and dedicate our food to the service of life.

Nirvana - Potatoes With Yogurt

Nirvana, means liberation. The combination of potato with yogurt, seasoned with the exotic spices, will definitely liberate your palate from all limitations. It is a nirvana for the palate. Taste for yourself how a simple potato can create rapture for your taste buds. Cook!

Preparation time: 25 minutes.

Serves 4-6.

2 lbs. small potatoes (scrubbed or peeled)

2 tbsp. ghee (1 tbsp. for potatoes, 1 tbsp. for spices)

1-2 fresh green chilli (seeded and cut crosswise), optional

1 tsp. garam masala

1 tsp. roasted ground cumin

1 tbsp. fresh ginger root (grated)

1 tsp. sea salt

1/4 tsp. ground dried red pepper (optional)

1 tsp. turmeric

1 cup yogurt

1 cup water

2 tbsp. fresh coriander leaves (chopped)

1. Boil potatoes for 15 minutes or till ready, then drain.
2. Heat 1 tbsp. ghee, add potatoes and fry till golden brown.
3. In a separate saucepan heat 1 tbsp. ghee.
4. Add chilli and the rest of the spices, stir well.
5. Add yogurt mixed with water, bring to boil and add potatoes.
6. Stir, cover, reduce the heat and cook for 5 more minutes.
7. Sprinkle with coriander leaves, garam masala and serve with rice.

Entree De La Paradise -
Green Papaya

Columbus called papaya "The Fruit of Paradise". It is not only exotic, it is curative. Papaya empowers the body. It adds frolic to your life and awakens your senses.

Preparation time: 20 minutes

Serves 4-6

1 tbsp. ghee

2 red dried chilli (optional)

2 bay leaves

1 tsp. punch phoron (see page 44)

4 medium potatoes (peeled and cubed)

1 green medium papaya, about 2 lb. (peeled and cubed)

1 tsp. turmeric

1/2 tsp. asafoetida

1 tsp. sea salt

1 tbsp. fresh ginger root (grated)

1 1/2 cup water

1. Heat ghee, add chilli, bay leaves and sizzle till brown.
2. Add panch phoron and sizzle till they pop.
3. Add potatoes, fry till golden brown.
4. Add papaya, turmeric, asafoetida, sea salt, ginger and stir well.
5. Add water, cover, lower the heat and cook till ready.
6. Serve hot with plain rice, or toasted bread.

Heavens Hash Brown -
Pumpkin And Potato

When you have to cook a fast dinner, cook Heavens Hash Brown. Just two vegetables and rice will give you a complete meal. It is sweet and delicious. Try it. It has everything your body needs.

Preparation time: 20 minutes.
Serves 4-6.

1 tbsp. ghee
1 dried red chilli (optional)
2 bay leaves
1/2 tsp. brown mustard seeds
1/2 tsp. kalonji (onion seeds)
4 medium potatoes (sliced like french fries)
1 lb. pumpkin (sliced like french fries)
1/2 tsp. turmeric
1 tsp. sea salt
2 tbsp. fresh ginger (grated)
1/2 cup water

1. Heat ghee, add red chilli, bay leaves and sizzle till brown.
2. Add mustard, kalonji and sizzle till they pop.
3. Add potatoes, fry till golden brown.
4. Add pumpkin, turmeric, sea salt and ginger.
5. Stir all ingredients well.
6. Add water, cover and cook till ready.
7. Serve hot with plain rice or toasted bread.

Fast Food For The Gods -
Rice With Vegetables

An easy, effortless and enjoyable way for body and mind empowerment. A very tasty, sattvic, light dish. A must for people who have tendency towards spiritual practices and meditation. It is a complete sumptuous meal by itself. A fast and delicious food for the sages.

Preparation time: 30 minutes.
Serves 4-6.

2 cups rice
1 small cauliflower (cut)
2 potatoes (cubed)
2 sweet potatoes (cubed)
6 cups water
1 tsp. sea salt
Ghee to taste

1. Combine rice, cauliflower, potatoes, sweet potatoes and water in a large pot.
2. Bring to boil, lower heat, cover and cook for 20 minutes.
3. Add salt. Do not let it dry. Keep consistency like porridge.
4. Serve hot. Add ghee to taste.

Sages Delight -
Rice and Pea Pulao

Sages love good food. Their dishes are simple, fast to cook and easy to digest. Sages Delight, together with the lentil soup (dal) and some green vegetables, makes a full meal.

Preparation time: 20 minutes.

Serves 4-6.

1 tbsp. ghee

1-2 green chilli (optional)

1 tsp. mustard seeds

1 tsp. cumin seeds

2 cups basmati rice

6 cups water

2 cups green peas

1 tsp. sea salt

1 tsp. turmeric

1. Heat ghee, add green chilli, mustard seeds and cumin seeds.
2. When seeds start to pop, add rice, water, peas, sea salt and turmeric.
3. Bring to boil, lower the heat, cover and cook for 20 minutes.

Divine Tenderness - Kitchari

A one-pot delicious and complete meal for a master. A favourite dish of the gods and the most served food in the temples.

Preparation time: 45 minutes. Serves 4-6.

2 cups rice
1/2 cup mung dal
1 small cauliflower (cut)
1 potato (cubed)
2 cups Indian pumpkin (cubed)
7 cups water
1 tsp. turmeric
1 tsp. sea salt
1 tbsp. ghee
1-2 dried red chilli (optional)
1/2 tsp. mustard seeds
1/2 tsp. cumin seeds
1/2 tsp. ajwan seeds
1/2 tsp. fenugreek seeds
1/2 tsp. asafoetida
1 tbsp. fresh ginger root (grated)
2 tbsp. coriander leaves (chopped)

1. In a large pot combine rice, dal, cauliflower, pumpkin, potato and water.
2. Bring to boil, add turmeric, salt, lower heat, cover and cook for 30 minutes.
3. At the end of cooking, heat the ghee in a small frying pan, add chilli, mustard, cumin, ajwan, fenugreek and sizzle till they pop.
4. Add asafoetida and ginger.
5. Add spice mixture to rice and dal, mix and cook till ready.
6. Garnish with coriander leaves. Eat hot with raitas, or chutney.

For The Busy Angels -
Rice And Yogurt

Just right for the busy "angel" for a fast and easy lunch or dinner.

Preparation time: 5-10 minutes.
Serves 4-6.

2 tbsp. ghee
1-2 dried red chilli (optional)
1/2 tsp. brown mustard seeds
1/2 tsp. cumin seeds
4 cups rice (cooked basmati rice)
1/4 tsp. black pepper (ground)
2 cups yogurt
1/4 tsp. turmeric
1 tsp. sea salt
2 tbsp. fresh coriander leaves (chopped)

1. Heat the ghee, add red chilli, mustard, cumin and sizzle till they pop.
2. Add cooked rice, salt and black pepper.
3. Stir well till rice becomes hot.
4. Remove from heat.
5. Mix turmeric with yogurt and pour over the rice.
6. Garnish with fresh coriander leaves. Serve hot.

CHAPTER 9

THE WATER OF LIFE
FOR BODY AND SOUL

Soups

The base of our soups is lentils, which are also called dal. They are the main source of protein in our diet. In combination with rice, or bread, lentils will provide you with an excellent source of protein.

Smaller lentils are faster cooking and easier to digest. Our favourites are Mung dal (small yellow lentils which may also be called split mung beans), and Musoor dal (small red lentils). Lentils are well known for their nourishing and strengthening benefits which may be applied to the convalescent as well as to the person in good health.

For best results cook dal fully or until it softens and breaks up - better to do it in the pot, than in the stomach. When it is well cooked it will be less likely to cause gas.

The most important factor in cooking dal is to add the herbs and spices according to the Phoron technique (see page 45). Follow the path of our recipes and bring the vital force of nature into your life. "Drink the Water of Life freely".

Hot Surprise -
Black Eyed Bean Soup

A very satisfying dish which will warm up your body and stimulate your senses. Together with plain rice or toasted bread, it will give you a complete protein meal.

Preparation time: 45 minutes.
Serves 4-6.

2 cups black eyed beans (soaked overnight)

10 cups water

2 tbsp. ghee

2 dried red chilli (optional)

2 bay leaves

1 tsp. cumin seeds

1 cinnamon stick

4 cardamom pods

1 tsp. ground turmeric

1/2 tsp. ground red chilli powder (optional)

2 tomatoes (chopped)

1 tsp. sea salt

2 tbsp. fresh ginger root (grated)

1 tsp. roasted ground cumin

2 tbsp. fresh coriander leaves (chopped)

1. Soak beans overnight, change water and bring to a boil.
2. Lower the heat, cover, and simmer till tender.
3. Heat the ghee in a saucepan, add chilli, bay leaves and sizzle till brown.
3. Add the rest of the ingredients, mix well, and sizzle for two minutes.
4. Add the spices to beans, mix well, and simmer for 5 more minutes.
5. Garnish with coriander leaves.
6. Serve hot with rice or bread.

Warm Affection -
Small Split Peas (Channa Dal)

A great offering for your body and soul. Nourishing and cleansing, building and energizing. It is low in fat and high in fibre. A great source of protein and iron.

Preparation time: 45 minutes.
Serves 4-6.

1 cup channa dal (soaked overnight)
10 cups water
1 tbsp. ghee
2 dried red chilli (optional)
2 bay leaves
1 cinnamon stick
3 green cardamom pods
1 tsp. turmeric
1 tsp. cumin
1 tbsp. fresh ginger root (grated)
1 tsp. sea salt
2 tbsp. raisins
2 tbsp. fresh coriander leaves (chopped)

1. Soak channa dal overnight, change water, bring to a boil, skim, lower the heat and cook until soft.
2. Heat the ghee in a separate pan, add chilli, bay leaves and sizzle till brown.
4. Add the rest of the ingredients including raisins and stir fry for one minute.
5. Add spice mixture to dal.
6. Simmer for 5 more minutes.
6. Garnish with fresh coriander, serve hot with rice, potatoes and vegetables.

Potent Power - Split Mung Beans With Vegetables
Yellow Lentils #1

Traditionally called Mung Dal Torchere. A meal by itself. Has everything to nourish and rejuvenate. Serve with plain rice to double the power and have a complete protein meal.

Preparation time: 50 minutes. Serves 4-6.

1 cup mung dal

15 cups water

3 potatoes (cubed)

1 sweet potato (cubed)

2 cups green peas

1 small cauliflower (cut into florets)

2 tbsp. ghee

1-2 dried red chilli (optional)

2 bay leaves

1 tsp. cumin

1 tsp. anise

4 medium fresh tomatoes (minced)

1 tsp. sea salt

1 tsp. turmeric

2 tbsp. fresh ginger root (grated)

1/2 tsp. asafoetida

2 tbsp. fresh coriander leaves (chopped)

1/2 roasted ground cumin

1. Bring mung dal to a boil, skim and cook for 30 minutes.
2. Add potatoes, sweet potatoes, green peas, cauliflower and cook till tender.
3. Heat the ghee, add chilli, bay leaves and sizzle till brown.
4. Add cumin, anise, and sizzle for few seconds.
5. Add tomatoes, salt, turmeric, ginger, asafoetida, saute for 2 minutes and add spice mixture to the dal.
6. Before the end of cooking, add coriander leaves, roasted ground cumin and serve hot with rice.

Power Of The Earth - Split Mung Beans With Vegetables
Yellow Lentils #2

You can make numerous varieties of this dish by changing the ingredients and adding your favourite vegetables. Try different combinations to create an ecstatic taste for your palate. The Power Of The Earth, dal and plain rice or bread - all you need to conquer the world.

Preparation time: - 50 minutes. Serves 4-6.

1 cup mung dal

10 cups water

2 potatoes (cubed)

1 sweet potato (cubed)

1 tbsp. ghee

2 dried red chilli (optional)

2 bay leaves

1 tsp. cumin seeds

1 tsp. fenugreek

1 tsp. fennel

4 medium fresh tomatoes (minced)

1 tsp. sea salt

1 tsp. turmeric

2 tbsp. fresh ginger root (grated)

1/2 tsp. asafoetida

1 bunch spinach (minced)

2 tbsp. coriander leaves (chopped)

1. Bring lentils to boil, skim and cook for 30 minutes.
2. Add potatoes, sweet potato and cook till tender.
3. In a small pot heat the ghee, add chilli and bay leaves, sizzle till brown.
4. Add cumin, fenugreek, fennel and sizzle for 10 seconds.
5. Add tomatoes, salt, turmeric, ginger, asafoetida, saute for 2 minutes and add spice mixture to the dal.
6. Add spinach and simmer for 2 more minutes.
7. Garnish with coriander leaves. Serve hot with rice or bread.

The Body's Delight - Musoor Beans
Red Lentils

This warm and satisfying dish is a source of power and strength. The broth itself will strengthen the weak and add energy to the warrior. The Body's Delight is light and nourishing, easy to digest and cooks faster than other lentils. Combined with rice, or toasted bread, it makes a complete protein meal for lunch or dinner.

Preparation time: 40 minutes. Serves 4-6.

1 cup red lentils

10 cups water

1 tbsp. ghee

1-2 dried red chilli (optional)

2 bay leaves

1/2 tsp. cumin seeds

1/2 tsp. fennel seeds

1/4 tsp. kalonji

1/4 tsp. fenugreek seeds

1/4 tsp. black mustard seeds

2 fresh tomatoes (minced)

1 tsp. sea salt

1 tsp. turmeric

1 tbsp. fresh ginger root (grated)

1/2 tsp. asafoetida

2 tbsp. fresh coriander leaves (chopped)

1. Bring lentils to the boil, lower heat and cook till tender.
2. In a small pot heat the ghee, add chillies and bay leaves and sizzle till brown.
3. Add cumin, fennel, kalonji, fenugreek, mustard seeds and sizzle till they pop.
4. Add tomatoes, salt, turmeric, ginger, asafoetida, saute for 2 minutes and add spice mixture to the dal.
5. Add coriander leaves and serve with rice or bread.

CHAPTER 10

THE GIFT OF HEAVEN AND EARTH

Rice

Rice is a main dish in this power program of cooking, as opposed to the common practice, where rice is a side dish along with other vegetables. Here rice is the foundation of the meal.

Rice is nourishing. It's qualities can fill volumes. It is the food for the gods. Both the ancient Chinese and the culture of the Sub-Continent of India have been eating rice this way from time immemorial.

Rice by itself has one of the highest quantities of absorbable protein. It balances body and mind. Make rice the basis of your meal.

There are many kinds of rice. We recommend Basmati rice because it is healthy, tasty and not par boiled. It is usually sun dried and is delicious to eat by itself with a touch of ghee.

Basmati rice is now available in most major supermarkets. It is grown on the terraced slopes and plains of the Himalayas, nurtured by the ancient mystical rivers Ganges and Jamuna. Translated, Basmati rice means "Fragrant pearl". Listen to the song of the Fragrant Pearl - this is what Basmati rice tells you:

The Song Of Myself -
Basmati Rice (Fragrant Pearl)

I was born on the Himalayas slopes,
Nurtured by the melting snow,
And breast fed by the sky
With the showers of the water of life.
And danced with the wind,
And reached up to the Sun,
That glistened all colours
Against the towering peaks.
I absorbed the fragrance of the Earth.
And now I am in your home.

I have brought power, strength and nourishment,
So that your body can harbour your soul
To romance with life.
To reach out for excellence.
To give vitality to your being.
To pour out fragrance.
To empower you,
And engulf you in ecstasy.
I will be immersed in you.
And rapture will be - the very essence.
Come, Take me.
And Romance The Stove.

Basmati Rice.

Here we give you some pointers to remember, when you cook the rice dishes that follow. When you are not sure, refer back to these pointers to get the best results.

Seven Secrets For Cooking Rice

Rice is the staple, the basic dish for lunch or dinner. We eat it, usually, once a day with lentils, or green vegetables and bread. It provides us with the required daily intake of proteins, vitamins and minerals.

Basmati rice is the fastest rice to cook and the easiest to digest. Grown on the slopes of Himalayas, it is lighter than other kinds of rice and more nutritious. Here are the seven secrets for cooking rice:

1. Wash rice a minimum of three times.
2. Use 2 cups of water to cook 1 cup of rice.
3. Drain rice well before sauteeing.
4. Saute rice in clarified butter before cooking. It keeps the grains from becoming mushy.
5. If you need to add more water, stir rice well to keep from sticking.
6. Cook rice till soft, but firm.
7. Mix gently with a fork to prevent grains from breaking.

The Gift Of Heaven And Earth - Plain Rice

Nothing tastes like plain rice flavoured with a touch of liquid gold - ghee. It goes with every constitution, with every mood, with all variations of the weather and is a perfect accompaniment to every dish. It is a true gift of Heaven and Earth.

Preparation time: 15 -20 minutes.
Serves 4-6.

2 cups rice
4 cups water
1 tsp. ghee for each serving, or to taste
sea salt to taste
fresh ground pepper to taste (optional)

1. Place rice in a medium pot and wash well.
2. Add water and bring to boil.
3. Lower the heat, do not cover and simmer till ready.
4. Serve with any food, or by itself.

A Meal For A Conqueror -
Pulao

Pulao is an excellent dish for entertaining and parties. It looks beautiful on the table and tastes simply delicious. It could be a meal by itself. To enhance the taste of pulao, serve it with cucumber raita (see page 90) or any other unsweetened yogurt dish.

Preparation time: 20 minutes.

Serves 4-6.

2 tbsp. ghee (1 tbsp. for rice, 1 tbsp. for spices)

2 cups rice

2 cups green peas (fresh or frozen)

5 cups water

1/2 tsp. mustard seeds

1/2 tsp. cumin seeds

10 cashews (chopped)

1 cup raisins

1/2 tsp. turmeric

1 tsp. sea salt

2 tbsp. coriander leaves (chopped)

1. Heat 1 tbsp. ghee, add rice (washed and drained).
2. Stir for 2 minutes, till coated with ghee.
3. Add green peas, water and bring to boil.
4. Lower heat, cover and cook till ready.
5. Uncover and cool cooked rice.
6. Heat 1 tbsp. ghee in a skillet, add mustard and cumin seeds, sizzle till they pop.
7. Add cashews, raisins, turmeric and salt.
8. Add cooked rice, peas and stir for two more minutes.
9. Garnish with coriander leaves. Serve hot.

Joy Of Life -
Spicy Fried Rice (Not Spicy Hot)

Preparation time: 20 minutes.

Serves 4-6.

2 tbsp. ghee

2 dried red chilli (optional)

2 bay leaves

1 tsp. cumin seeds

1 cinnamon stick

4 cardamom pods

5 cloves

1 tsp. turmeric

2 cups basmati rice (washed and drained)

1 tsp. sea salt

4 cups boiling water

2 tbsp. coriander leaves (chopped)

1. Heat the ghee, add dried red chilli, bay leaves and sizzle till brown.
2. Add cumin, cinnamon, cardamom, cloves, turmeric and sizzle for a few seconds.
3. Add rice, salt and stir till lightly golden.
4. Add boiling water, bring to a boil, lower heat to minimum, cover and cook for 20 minutes.
4. When all the water has been absorbed, remove from heat.
5. Remove cinnamon stick, cardamom pods, cloves and chilli before serving.
6. Garnish with coriander leaves. Serve hot.

Prologue -
Fried Rice And Cauliflower

Preparation time: 20 minutes.

Serves 4-6.

2 tbsp. ghee

1 dried red chilli (optional)

3 bay leaves

4 cardamom pods

1 tsp. cumin seeds

2 cinnamon sticks

1 cauliflower (cut into florets)

1 tsp. turmeric

1 tsp. sea salt

1 tbsp. fresh ginger root (grated)

2 tbsp. coriander leaves (chopped)

2 cups rice

5 cups water

1. Heat ghee, add chilli, bay leaves and sizzle till brown.
2. Add cardamom, cumin, cinnamon and sizzle for 30 seconds.
3. Add cauliflower and stir for 1 minute.
4. Add washed and drained rice, turmeric, salt, ginger, fresh coriander.
5. Stir for 1 minute and mix spices well.
6. Add 5 cups of water and bring to boil.
7. Lower heat, cover and cook for 15-20 min. until water has evaporated.
8. Remove cinnamon sticks, cardamom pods and chilli before serving.
9. Garnish with coriander leaves, fluff and serve hot.

CHAPTER 11

THE LOVE OF VENUS

Vegetables

Vegetables are medicine, the very foundation of life on the planet Earth. From them comes our vitality and physical strength.

They empower the Mars activity of man, create tonicity of the muscles. Vegetables are venusian. Venus is the spirit of the kitchen gardens and their fertility.

All grains, roots, flowers, herbs, seeds and fruits are the progeny of the romance between the Sun and the Earth. Some vegetables mature in the air above ground while others perform their magic unseen, below the surface, in the realm of the Moon.

Let us give some further attention to the relationship between the abundant gifts that Mother Earth in her generosity provides for the nourishment of her children and the custodial role that we need to play as grateful recipients of that bounty.

In the Bible, Eden was a garden. "And the Lord God took the man, and put him into the garden of Eden to dress it and keep it." (Genesis 2:15) "And God said, Behold I have given you every herb bearing seed, which is upon the face of all the earth, and every tree, in the which is the fruit of a tree yielding seed; to you it shall be for meat". (Genesis 1:29)

And so, it is from the vegetable kingdom of growing things that we harvest our food, our medicine, our health and our wealth.

In the mystic realm once again, let us give homage to Venus as the morning and evening star in the twilight sky, whose light reaches Earth and inspires all vegetation with her beauty and her radiance.

Let me reveal the seven secrets for cooking vegetables.

Seven Secrets For Cooking Vegetables

You can create numerous dishes when you know the secrets of cooking vegetables. The following tips will show you how to transform simple vegetables into sumptuous meals.

1. The first secret lies in spices, in knowing how to combine different spices in certain proportions; this information is given in every recipe.

2. The second secret lies in the right combination of vegetables with other foods.

3. The third secret lies in eating vegetables hot and well cooked. We do not eat raw carrot, cauliflower, or broccoli. Why abuse your stomach when the pot can do the work?

4. The fourth secret lies in selecting vegetables. Naturally grown food is better than chemically pumped vegetables.

5. The fifth secret lies in eating vegetables (if it is possible), grown in your area.

6. The sixth secret is the Phoron technique. This is how to do it:

   a) Heat clarified butter (ghee), or vegetable oil.

   b) Add spices and sizzle them in the order required.

   c) Add vegetables and saute them in spices.

   d) Add some liquid, water, or yogurt.

   e) Cover, lower the heat and cook till ready.

7. The seventh secret lies in avoiding deep fried, canned and frozen food. Why? Because fresh vegetables are tastier and have all of their food value intact for promoting strength, joy and longevity.

Exotic Serenade -
Spinach And Swiss Chard

Spinach and swiss chard help to heal the liver and immune system. They are very rich in minerals and vitamins. They are good for the skin, eyes and bladder. Raw spinach and swiss chard are hard to digest. They must be slightly cooked to assist digestion and the process of elimination.

Preparation time: 10 minutes.

Serves 4-6.

1 tbsp. ghee

1 dried red chilli (optional)

2 bay leaves

1 tsp. fennel seeds

1 tsp. cumin seeds

1/4 tsp. mustard seeds

1 bunch spinach (cut)

1 bunch swiss chard (cut)

2 tbsp. fresh ginger root (grated)

2 tbsp. coriander leaves (chopped)

1/2 tsp. sea salt or to taste

1 tsp. turmeric

1. Heat ghee, add red chilli, bay leaves and sizzle till brown.
2. Add fennel, cumin, mustard seeds and sizzle for 15 seconds.
3. Add spinach, swiss chard, ginger, coriander, salt, turmeric and stir.
4. Lower the heat, cover and cook for 10 min., or till tender.
5. Stir again to mix all spices well.
6. Serve hot with rice.

Song Of The Sun -
Swiss Chard And Potatoes

Preparation time: 20 minutes.

Serves 4-6.

1 tbsp. ghee

2 dried red chilli (optional)

2 bay leaves

1 tsp. cumin seeds

1 tsp. brown mustard seeds

4 large potatoes

1 tbsp. poppy seeds

1/2 tsp. asafoetida

2 bunches swiss chard (cut)

2 tbsp. fresh ginger root (grated)

1 tsp. turmeric

1/2 tsp. sea salt, or to taste

2 tbsp. coriander leaves (chopped)

1. Heat ghee, add red chilli, bay leaves and sizzle till brown.
2. Add cumin, mustard seeds and sizzle for a few seconds.
3. Add potatoes and stir fry till slightly golden.
4. Add poppy seeds, asafoetida and stir.
5. Add swiss chard, ginger, turmeric, salt, cover tight and cook for five minutes.
6. Lower heat to medium, stir well, and cook for 10 minutes.
7. Garnish with coriander leaves.
8. Serve hot with rice, or bread.

Echo Of The Moon -
Spicy Eggplant (Not Spicy Hot)

Preparation time: 15 minutes.

Serves 4-6.

2 tbsp. ghee

1 tsp. cumin seeds

4 long Indian eggplants-also called Japanese eggplant

(cut length-wise first, then in half)

1/4 tsp. sea salt

1/4 tsp. freshly ground black pepper (optional)

1. Heat the ghee in a large frying pan.
2. Add cumin seeds and sizzle for 30 seconds.
3. Add eggplant slices and fry on both sides until golden brown.
3. Cover, lower the heat to simmer for 15 minutes, or till soft.
4. Add salt and pepper.
5. Serve hot with rice.
6. Cold eggplant is an excellent alternative filling for our sandwich, called "A Date With The Taste Buds" (see page 86).

Whisper Of The Wind -
Sizzled Potatoes And Cauliflower

Preparation time: 20 minutes.

Serves 4-6.

1 tbsp. ghee

2 dried red chilli (optional)

3 bay leaves

1 tsp. mustard seeds (brown)

1 tsp. cumin seeds

4 potatoes (cubed)

1 medium cauliflower (cut in small pieces)

4 small tomatoes

1 tsp. turmeric

1/2 tsp. asafoetida

1 tbsp. fresh ginger root (grated)

1 tsp. sea salt

1 cup water

2 tbsp. fresh coriander leaves (chopped)

1. Heat ghee, add red chilli, bay leaves and sizzle till brown.
2. Add mustard seeds, cumin seeds and sizzle till they pop.
3. Add potatoes, stir and saute till slightly golden.
4. Add cauliflower, tomatoes, turmeric, asafoetida, ginger, salt and stir for 2 minutes.
5. Add water, bring to a boil, lower heat to medium and cook for 10 minutes, or till ready.
7. Sprinkle with coriander before serving.

Accompaniment 1 -
Potato With Dill And Coriander

Preparation time: 20 minutes.

Serves 4-6.

1 tbsp. ghee

1-2 dried red chilli (optional)

1 tsp. cumin seeds

1/2 tsp. fennel seeds

1 bunch green onions (chopped)

1 tbsp. fresh ginger root (grated)

4 medium potatoes (cut into 4 pieces, boiled)

1/2 tsp. turmeric

2 fresh tomatoes (chopped)

2 tbsp. fresh dill (chopped)

2 tbsp. fresh coriander leaves (chopped)

1/4 tsp. black pepper (optional)

1/2 tsp. sea salt or to taste

1. Heat ghee, add red chilli, sizzle till brown.
2. Add cumin, fennel and sizzle for 15 seconds.
3. Add green onions, ginger and sizzle for 1 minute.
4. Add cooked potato, turmeric, tomatoes and stir well.
5. Add dill, coriander, black pepper and salt to taste.
6. Mix well to blend the spices.
7. Serve hot with rice and vegetables.

Accompaniment 2 -
Forget Me Not (Eggplant Spread)

Preparation time: 20 minutes.
Serves 4-6.

2 large eggplants
1/2 tsp. sea salt
2 tbsp. sunflower oil
1/4 tsp. black pepper
2 green chilli (optional, finely chopped)

1. Place the eggplant under a pre-heated grill or microwave for 20 minutes turning frequently until soft.
2. Peel cooked eggplant and mash with fork.
3. Add green chilli, sea salt, sunflower oil, black pepper and mix well.
4. Serve with rice or bread. An excellent filling for our sandwich called "A Date With The Taste Buds" (see page 86).

Accompaniment 3 -
Tomato And Cucumber Tango

This "Tomato And Cucumber Tango", refreshed by lime juice is very beneficial to the heart, throat and voice.

2 large tomatoes (chopped)
2 large cucumbers (peeled and chopped)
1 large lime (juice)
2 green chilli (optional, finely chopped)
2 tbsp. fresh coriander leaves (chopped)
1/2 tsp. sea salt or to taste
1/4 tsp. black ground pepper

1. Mix all ingredients together in a bowl. Cover and chill.
2. A great accompaniment for lunch or dinner.

CHAPTER 12

THE FAST FOOD OF PARADISE

When Pressed For Time,
Try These Sandwiches

A sandwich is composed of the unity of two pieces of bread attached with the ecstasy of filling. Perhaps, we could express it in a more poetic way by replacing the filling with love. This is romance. This is health. This is joy and ecstasy - the celebration of mind and body, the house of the soul.

Enjoy these sandwiches - let the taste buds blossom in laughter, and flood your mouth with the juices of life; sensual adventures for the tongue.

A Date With The Taste Buds -
When This Date Comes All Of A Sudden

Bite softly. The sensation will awaken the taste buds from slumber. Be sure to enjoy every bite and celebrate the body.

Preparation time: 5 minutes.

Warning: Pre-Prepare your eggplant. These dates come all of a sudden (see recipes on pages 82 and 85).

Bread of your choice (toasted)
Eggplant (see our recipes as per pages above)
Sea salt to taste
Freshly ground Black pepper to taste
Fresh coriander leaves (chopped)

1. Toast the bread.
2. Place eggplant-the filling (love), on toast.
3. Add sea salt, pepper and coriander leaves to taste.
4. Cover with another toast and eat.

The Celestial Sandwich - The Paradox Of Heaven

Eat this sandwich with a quiet mind, and you may hear the angels sing.

Preparation time: 5 minutes
English muffin (toasted)
Avocado (sliced)
Cucumber (peeled and sliced)
Tomato (sliced)
Alfalfa sprouts
Fresh coriander leaves (finely chopped)
Sea salt to taste
Fresh ground black pepper to taste

1. Toast muffin till golden brown.
2. Let it cool for 1 minute.
3. Add avocado, cucumber, tomatoes, Alfalfa sprouts and coriander leaves.
4. Add salt and pepper to taste.

Sandwich For A Hungry Monk

Enjoy, but remind yourself that there is more to life than eating.

Preparation Time: 10 minutes.
4 Pita breads
4 Tomatoes (chopped)
1 sweet fresh red pepper (chopped)
1/2 tsp. sea salt
1/2 tsp. ground black pepper
2 tbsp. fresh coriander (chopped)
1 cup havarti cheese (grated)

1. Heat oven to 450 F.
2. Place the bread on the oven tray and add tomatoes, red pepper, salt and pepper.
3. Top it with fresh coriander leaves.
4. Add cheese to cover all vegetables and bake until cheese melts.
5. Serve hot with tea of your choice.

Post Romance Sandwich -
Have It Ready Before The Loving Begins

Warning: The cycle can begin faster than you know.

Preparation time: 10 minutes.

1 avocado (mashed)
1 tomato (chopped)
1 cucumber (chopped)
1 fresh green chilli (chopped), optional
Sea salt to taste
Ground black pepper to taste
Muesli bread (toasted)

1. Mix all vegetables together.
2. Add salt and pepper to taste.
3. Toast muesli bread.
4. Spread mashed vegetable mixture on the toast, cover with another
   slice of toast and enjoy.

CHAPTER 13

THE ADVENTURE OF LIFE

The Exotic Yogurt Salads (Raita)
Where Vegetables Are The Dressing

For Electrifying And Intensifying The Taste Buds
Feel How They Blossom

Raita is a potent addition to the flavouring of food. It helps the digestive process. It cleanses the tongue of the coating of the previous bite, to welcome with zest the next bite.

It is a salad in reverse. Yogurt is the salad. The vegetables are the dressing.

Discover the greater joy of eating.

The ecstasy of the tongue needs to be controlled.

Nirvana approaches...

Mild And Soothing -
Cucumber Raita

A delightful addition with lunch or dinner. This dish helps digestion. It is taken between bites to enhance the taste and clear the palate to become ready for the next bite.

Preparation time: 10 minutes.

2 cups yogurt

1 cup cucumber (peeled and grated)

1 tsp. fresh ginger root (peeled and grated)

1/4 tsp. turmeric

1/2 tsp. roasted ground cumin

1/2 tsp. sea salt

1/4 tsp. black pepper (ground)

2 tbsp. finely chopped coriander leaves

1-2 green chillies (chopped, optional)

1. Mix yogurt until smooth.
2. Add the rest of ingredients.
3. Mix well together.
4. Chill and serve as a side dish or garnish for rice, breads and vegetables.

Liberates And Awakens -
Potato Raita

Enjoyed by many. This dish liberates and awakens the taste buds. You can hear the laughter of the food in your body.

Preparation time: 20 minutes.

2 cups boiled potatoes (peeled and diced)

1/2 tsp. sea salt

2 tbsp. fresh dill (chopped)

1 tsp. roasted ground cumin

1-2 green chillies (chopped, optional)

2 tbsp. fresh scallions (chopped, optional)

1/4 tsp. ground black pepper

2 cups yogurt

1. Mix boiled and diced potatoes with all the ingredients except yogurt.
2. Blend yogurt in a bowl until smooth and add to potatoes.
4. Mix well and serve as a side dish.

Renews And Rejuvenates -
Beet and Carrot Raita

As an accompaniment with lunch or dinner, it enhances the flavour of food and stimulates the taste buds. It is taken between bites to clean the palate so it is ready to enjoy the next bite. It helps in digestion, renews and rejuvenates the body.

Preparation time: 20 minutes.

2 cups yogurt

2 cups boiled beets (peeled and diced)

1 cup boiled carrots (peeled and diced)

1/2 tsp. sea salt

2 tsp. honey, or maple syrup

1-2 green chillies (chopped, optional)

1/4 roasted ground coriander seeds

2 tbsp. chopped coriander leaves

1 tbsp. ghee

1 tsp. brown mustard seeds

1. Blend yogurt in a bowl until smooth.
2. Add cooked and diced beets and carrots as well as the remaining ingredients, except ghee and mustard seeds.
3. Heat ghee, add mustard seeds and sizzle until they start to pop.
4. Remove from stove and add to yogurt mixture.
5. Mix well. Serve as a side dish.

CHAPTER 14

THE ENHANCED ADVENTURE OF LIFE

Relishes and Chutneys

To Bring Sparkle And Refinement To The Senses

Relishes/Chutneys are usually served to add distinctive flavour and piquant taste to the food. Chutneys heat your palate, when raitas cool it off. They stimulate digestion. Relishes add a sparkle and refinement to your senses. They make your tongue tingle and move with enthusiasm and zest. Relishes make your meal a celebration, a feast of joy and a delight.

Excellent for one who loves adventures.

Relish what is before you!

Spice up your life!

A Cooling Touch -
Coriander Chutney

Adds piquantness and freshness to your food. Good with bread, rice dishes, vegetables and soups. A must for a Formal dinner.

Surprise your guests with the unique flavour of your personal touch. Enjoy the refreshing coolness in your mouth. Make eating an adventure.

Preparation time: 10 minutes.

2 bunches fresh coriander leaves

1/4 cup lemon/lime juice

1/2 cup tamarind sauce (see page 41)

1/2 cup water

4 tbsp. fresh ginger root (grated)

1 tsp. sea salt

1 tsp. honey or 4 dates (optional)

2-4 green chillies (optional)

1. Blend all ingredients together until you have a smooth paste.
2. Store in jars with caps.
3. Keep refrigerated (good for about one week).

A Touch Of The Divine - Basil Chutney

Cooked basil could be overwhelming, but fresh basil adds to foods a heavenly taste of the Divine presence. Good with breads, rice dishes and vegetables. Excellent for people who want to increase their memory, practice meditation and spiritual work.

Feel the sublime presence. Make eating a spiritual quest.

Preparation time: 10 minutes.

2 bunches fresh basil leaves
7 tbsp. lemon/lime juice
4 tbsp. fresh ginger root (grated)
1 tsp. sea salt
2-4 green chillies (optional)
1/2 cup tamarind sauce (see page 41)
1/2 cup water

1. Blend all ingredients together until you have a smooth paste.
2. Keep refrigerated (good for about one week).

A Refining Touch -
Mint Chutney

A great stimulant in the art of eating. Best when used fresh. Helps digestive and nervous systems. Mint chutney has a cooling and soothing effect on body and mind.

Experience a refined sensation in your mouth: cultivate your gourmet taste buds.

Preparation time: 10 minutes.

2 bunches fresh mint leaves
7 tbsp. lemon/lime juice
4 tbsp. fresh ginger (grated)
1 tsp. sea salt
2-4 green chillies (optional)
1/2 cup tamarind sauce (see page 41)
1/2 cup water

1. Blend all ingredients together until you have a smooth paste.
2. Keep refrigerated (good for about one week)

A Spark Of Cool Fire -
Mint And Coriander Chutney

An excellent combination of herbs. Very effective for digestion and absorption of other foods. It helps to restore the body after colds, nervous tension and congestion. Good with grain dishes, vegetables and breads.

Feel a fountain of joyful sensations in your mouth. Let the sparkle of ecstasy start the cleansing fire in your body.

Preparation time: 10 minutes.

1 bunch of mint leaves

1 bunch of coriander leaves

7 tbsp. lemon juice

4 tbsp. fresh ginger root (grated)

1 tsp. sea salt

2-4 green chillies (optional)

1/2 cup tamarind sauce (see page 41)

1/2 cup water

1. Blend all ingredients together until you have a smooth paste.
2. Keep refrigerated (good for one week).

CHAPTER 15

THE ESSENCE (SOUL) OF THE HERBS

Hot Teas
For Enjoinment And Healing

Tea, in its most familiar form, has been made with the leaves of a tea plant, an evergreen shrub called "Camellia sinensis" and has originated manly in India and China. It is a drink made by infusing tea leaves in boiling water. Legend has it that the soul of the leaves was extracted by this process and by drinking the charged liquid, the soul of the drinker would be nourished through the agency of the nerves.

In the most recent years however, we have extended the range of our teas to include the infusing of herbs, seeds and spices in hot water, combining them with other ingredients and naming them after the major herb used.

So why not extract the essence, the spirit of other great herbs, seeds and spices and prepare a variety of ambrosia to suit the occasion.

A Cup Of Strength -
Fenugreek Tea: I Have Not Yet Begun To Fight

Breath and sex are the very essence of all things in this manifested universe. Fenugreek helps to strengthen both - the respiratory and reproductive systems.

Your friends and folks will want to know your secret - where you get your jubilant energy from, when the rest of the work force is fading away, craving for the lunch hour to arrive, you get your second wind.

Enjoy A Cup Of Strength. Live long, prosper and multiply!

Warning: Not recommended for pregnant women.

Soaking time: overnight.
Preparation time - 5 minutes.
Serves 4.

4 tsp. fenugreek seeds
4 cups water
honey (to taste)
lemon/lime (to taste)

1. Soak fenugreek seeds in 4 cups water overnight.
2. Boil the same water with the seeds for 5 minutes.
3. Strain, add honey and lemon/lime to taste.

A Cup Of Courage -
Ginger Tea: The Universal Medicine

A great stimulant during the latter part of the day or for people who burn the midnight oil. It is also a good starter in the morning for the warrior.

According to Ayurveda it is the best of all spices. It promotes power. The Oxford dictionary defines ginger as "spirit", "mettle". It helps strengthen the digestive and respiratory systems. It is a friend of the heart - a heart tonic. Try ginger tea to help headaches as well. It helps to develop stamina, tenacity and bravery.

Spice up your life with A Cup Of Courage. Live in this world of turmoil as calm and serene as a sage.

Preparation time - 5 to 15 minutes.
Serves 4.

4 cups water
2" fresh ginger root (chopped)
unpasteurized honey (to taste)
lemon/lime (to taste)

1. Bring water to a boil, add ginger.
2. Reduce heat and simmer for 5-15 minutes, depending on the strength that suites your taste.
3. Strain, add honey and lemon to taste.

A Cup Of Triumph -
Mind, Body and Spirit Balancing Tea

As you sip this tea the vibrations of the universe beats to your own rhythm. A Cup Of Triumph goes with everything. It contains herbs and spices that invigorate the essence of your being.

Serve A Cup Of Triumph with dignity and befriend all your guests. Drink this nectar and balance with the universe.

Preparation time - 5 to 15 minutes.

Serves 4.

4 cups water

2" fresh ginger root (sliced)

4 cardamom pods

4 cloves

1 cinnamon stick

lemon/lime (to taste)

unpasteurized honey (to taste)

1. Boil water, add all spices.
2. Reduce heat and simmer for 5-15 minutes, depending on the strength that suites your taste.
3. Strain, add honey and lemon.

A Cup Of Caring -
For Leisure And Enjoyment

A perfect tea to share with close friends or business associates.

Drink A Cup Of Caring with satisfaction. Feel the warmth and comfort of friendship.

Preparation time - 5 to 15 minutes.
Serves 4.

2 cups 2 % milk
2 cups water
4 cardamom pods
4 cloves
2" fresh ginger (sliced)
1 cinnamon stick
1/4 tsp. turmeric
unpasteurized honey (to taste)

1. Boil water and milk together, add all spices except turmeric and ginger.
2. Reduce heat and simmer for 5-15 minutes, depending on the strength that suites your taste.
3. Add turmeric, ginger and stir well.
4. Strain and add honey to taste.

A Cup Of Tranquility -
For Pleasant Dreams

A perfect tea before meditation or prayer. It enhances the intimate time with your own Self, when intellect and ego are put to rest and you are face to face with your own Soul.

Drink A Cup Of Tranquility with calmness. Feel the soothing, nourishing and loving presence of the Divine.

Preparation time - 5 to 15 minutes.
Serves 2.

1 cup milk 2%
1 cup water
1" fresh ginger (sliced)
1/8 tsp. turmeric
1/2 tsp. ghee (clarified butter, optional)
unpasteurized honey (to taste)

1. Bring milk and water to a boil, add ginger.
2. Reduce heat and simmer for 5-15 minutes, depending on the strength that suites your taste.
3. Add turmeric and ghee.
4. Stir, strain and add honey to taste.

A Cup Of Joy -
For Getting Impulse Power

Do you feel a bit sluggish, sleepy and tired? If so, the Cup Of Joy is right for you. Try it and get the impulse power.

Preparation time: 5 - 10 minutes.
Serves 2.

1 cup 2% milk
1 cup water
2 tsp. loose tea
1/2 tsp. garam masala (see page 42)
1 tsp. honey (optional)

1. Boil water and milk together with tea and spices.
2. Stir constantly.
3. Strain, add honey to taste and serve hot.

A Cup Of Awakening -
For Reaching The Stars At Warp Speed

Dynamite! Try it for breakfast or when you are losing speed. It works!

Preparation time: 5 - 10 minutes.
Serves 2.

1 cup 2% milk
1 cup water
1/2 tsp. garam masala (see page 42)
1/2 tsp. fresh ginger root (grated)
1/4 tsp. turmeric
1 tsp. honey (optional)

1. Boil water and milk.
2. When boiled well, add ginger, turmeric and spices.
3. Strain and add honey to taste.

COLD NOURISHING DRINKS

A Call Of The Tropics -
Banana Milk Shake With Spices

A great drink for breakfast with your favourite cereal.

Preparation time: 2 minutes.
Serves 2.

2 bananas
2 cups milk
1/4 tsp. garam masala (see page 42)

1. Blend all ingredients together in blender.
2. Drink right after it is made.

A Taste Of Paradise -
Mango Milk Shake

Delicious! Try it for breakfast with any cereal or by itself.

Preparation time: 2 minutes.
Serves 2.

2 ripe mangos
2 cups milk
1/8 tsp. ground cardamom seeds
2 tsp. raw sugar or honey (optional)

1. Blend all ingredients together in blender.
2. Drink right after it is made.

PART FOUR

CREATING ROMANCE

CHAPTER 16

THE FORMAL WAY

In this section you will find a series of menus for lunch and dinner along with a light breakfast and a snack.

These are pre-set menus. However, when you become more familiar with the nature of the dishes, you can create your own combinations toward a balanced diet, the enjoyment of eating, entertaining and staying healthy.

In part one of the book we have carefully given the medicinal values and particular characteristics of the spices and herbs we use in our cooking with the expectation that, in regard to health: "An ounce of prevention is worth a pound of cure." We practice this on a daily basis ourselves.

We have also given each dish an unusual name. There is a subtle purpose intended here. Apart from the entertainment value, these names will give your subconscious mind subliminal suggestions of health, joy and romance which in turn will manifest in your body and environment. Your attitude towards eating will evolve to a higher spiral. Even if you are sceptical now, after a short practice you will begin to share our feelings of celebration during meal times.

Just imagine, instead of having Swiss Chard and Spinach you will be serving "Exotic Serenade" with its blend of seasoning and spice. Instead of serving a cup of Ginger tea, you will offer "A Cup Of Courage"!

If you are artistically oriented and have an inclination towards a bit of flamboyancy, you could put these menus in your computer and print them out on a special menu format before serving meals to your family or friends or just for yourself - another addition of fun and romance in your entertaining.

We have found that having the menu prior to food being served adds a touch of class around the dinner table.

Try it! Create your own romance and celebrate living!

SEVEN DAYS OF MENUS

Day One

Breakfast

The Romantic's Delight -
Fresh Home Made Cheese (Paneer)

A Cup Of Joy -
For Getting Impulse Power

Lunch

The Divine Tenderness -
One Pot Meal (Kitchari)

A Cooling Touch -
Coriander Chutney

The Milk Of Human Kindness -
1/2 Cup Buttermilk Drink (Lassi)

Snack

Fresh Fruits

Dinner

The Potent Power -
Mung Bean Soup With Vegetables #1

The Paradoxical Waltz -
Potato With White Radish

Mild And Soothing -
Cucumber Raita

Day Two

Breakfast

Sandwich For A Hungry Monk

A Cup Of Strength -
The Fenugreek Tea: I Have Not Yet Begun To Fight

Lunch

A Meal For A Conqueror -
Pulao

The Power House -
Spinach And Potato

A Spark Of Cool Fire -
Mint And Coriander Chutney

Milk Of Human Kindness -
1/2 cup Buttermilk Drink (Lassi)

Snack

Fresh Fruits

Dinner

The Gift Of Heaven And Earth -
Plain Rice

Warm Affection -
Small Split Pea Soup

Renews And Rejuvenates -
Beet And Carrot Raita

Day Three

Breakfast

Choice Of Preferred Cereal

A Call Of The Tropics -
Banana Milk Shake With Spices

Lunch

Heavens Hash Brown -
Pumpkin And Potato

The Sages Delight -
Rice And Green Peas Pulao

A Touch Of The Divine -
Basil Chutney

The Milk Of Human Kindness -
1/2 cup Buttermilk Drink (Lassi)

Snack

10 Raw Almonds (Soaked Overnight)

Dinner

Hot Surprise -
Black Eyed Bean Soup

Accompaniment 3 -
Tomato And Cucumber Tango

Toasted Bread

Day Four

Breakfast

For The Busy Angels -
Rice And Yogurt

A Cup Of Courage -
The Ginger Tea

Lunch

The Exotica De Bengal -
Potato And Cabbage

Warm Affection -
Small Split Pea Soup

Toasted Unleavened Bread

The Milk Of Human Kindness -
1/2 Cup Buttermilk Drink (Lassi)

Snack

Fresh Fruits

Dinner

The Ultimate Tango -
Cottage Cheese With Green Peas

The Gift Of Heaven And Earth -
Plain Rice

A Refining Touch -
Mint Chutney

Day Five

Breakfast

Fresh Fruits

A Cup Of Triumph -
Mind, Body And Spirit Balancing Tea

Lunch

Fast Food For The Gods -
Rice With Vegetables
(One Pot Meal)

A Touch Of The Divine -
Basil Chutney

The Milk Of Human Kindness -
1/2 Cup Buttermilk Drink (Lassi)

Snack

Choice Of Favourite Nuts
(One Hand Full)

Dinner

Venus And Mars On A Plate -
Zucchini And Tomatoes

Liberates And Awakens -
Potato Raita

Toasted Bread

Day Six

Breakfast

The Romantic's Delight -
Fresh Home Made Cheese (Paneer)

A Cup Of Joy -
For Getting Impulse Power

Lunch

The Soothing Touch -
Okra and Potato

Accompaniment 3 -
Tomato And Cucumber Tango

Toasted Bread

Snack

Fresh Fruits

Dinner

The Gift Of Heaven And Earth -
Plain Rice

Entree De La Paradise -
Green Papaya

The Body's Delight -
Red Lentil Soup (Musoor Dal)

The Milk Of Human Kindness -
1/2 Cup Buttermilk Drink (Lassi)

Day Seven

Breakfast

Choice Of Hot Cereal

A Cup Of Awakening -
For Reaching The Stars At Warp Speed

Lunch

Nirvana -
Potato With Yogurt

The Celestial Sandwich -
The Paradox Of Heaven

Snack

Fresh Fruits

Dinner

Hindu Russi Bhai! Bhai! -
Not Just Another Cabbage Roll

The Joy Of Life -
Spicy Rice (Not Spicy Hot)

A Refining Touch -
Mint Chutney

The Milk Of Human Kindness -
1/2 Cup Buttermilk Drink (Lassi)

FORMAL DINNERS

The Philharmonic Symphony -
A Formal Dinner # 1

The Usher -
Unsweetened Organic Pure Grape Juice

Prologue -
Rice and Cauliflower

Exotic Serenade -
Spinach and Swiss Chard

The Body's Delight -
Red Lentils (Musoor Dal)

Accompaniment 1 -
Potato with Dill and Coriander

Accompaniment 2 -
Eggplant - Forget Me Not

Accompaniment 3 -
Tomato and Cucumber Tango

Served With
A Spark Of Cool Fire
And
The Milk Of Human Kindness

Quintessence-The Offering Of Power -
A Formal Dinner # 2

Joy Of Life -
Spicy Rice (Not Spicy Hot)

Song Of The Sun -
Swiss Chard And Potato

Echo Of The Moon -
Spicy Eggplant (Not Spicy Hot)

Whisper Of The Wind -
Sizzled Potatoes And Cauliflower

Power Of The Earth -
Split Mung Beans With Vegetables
(Yellow Lentil Soup #2)

Serve with
A Refining Touch
And
The Milk Of Human Kindness

About The Author

Samahria Ramsen is a romantic poet and an inspirational spiritual writer. She has a Master of Education degree. Her passion for knowledge and compassion for all aspects of life has prompted her to travel extensively in quest of the fulfilment of her ideals.

Even though she is a daughter of a physician she has not been immune to the unhealthy influence of improper diet and life style. She was brought up on a primarily meat and fish based diet. Over time, a number of factors including poor eating habits led to a deterioration in her health. Frequent sickness and the search for new doctors and drugs had become a familiar part of her existence.

After going through many traumatic experiences, she found herself in serious physical and emotional disharmony. Excruciating pain drove her to a new quest - to build a perfect body that was a suitable dwelling place for the soul.

Her new search took her to the far corners of the earth with little results until, at the fortunate moment, she met her true spiritual teacher. He taught her how to create a dynamic balance between the body, mind and soul. She also learned the ancients secrets of right eating and right thinking, which are inseparable twins. She learned that romancing the Self or the Soul is the only true romance.

She now realizes that old habits and non-productive ways of thinking often restrict us from living a full and enchanting life. She recommends that we adopt an open mind to the teaching that "health is wealth" and joyfully enter into the spirit of her book Romancing The Stove.

It is the heartfelt desire of the author that the knowledge and experience that she has gained from her teacher be shared with her readers as an invitation to a new adventure in creative living through cooking and eating for health.

ORDER FORM

A LIMITED NUMBER OF AUTOGRAPHED COPIES OF ROMANCING THE STOVE ARE AVAILABLE

YES, I want to order Romancing The Stove. Please send me ___ copies at $19.95 each plus $4.50 for the first copy and $1.50 for each additional copy to cover shipping and handling. I understand that my order may take from four to six weeks for delivery. Please address my order to:

Name
_____

Organization
_____

Address
_____

City/State/Zip
_____

My check or money order for $_____is enclosed.

Please make your check or money order payable to:

Omnilux® Communications Inc.

Mail your check with the order to the publisher:

Omnilux® Communications Inc.
PO Box #255,
Etobicoke 'A', Ontario, M9C 4V2

P.S.

For more information on the Romancing The Stove Program, products, herbs and spices, or if you want to share your experiences, recipes or stories with Mrs. Ramsen, please write to the above address.